Nerve

Michele T. Pato

Nerve

A Physician Turned Patient and Her
Courageous Recovery From Traumatic
Brain Injury

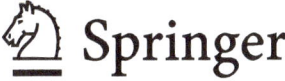 Springer

Michele T. Pato
Robert Wood Johnson Medical School
Rutgers, The State University of New Jersey
New Brunswick, NJ, USA

ISBN 978-3-031-33432-0   ISBN 978-3-031-33433-7   (eBook)
https://doi.org/10.1007/978-3-031-33433-7

This Springer imprint is published by the registered company Springer Nature Switzerland AG
The registered company address is: Gewerbestrasse 11, 6330 Cham, Switzerland

Paper in this product is recyclable.

The only way to live is by accepting each minute as an unrepeatable miracle.

—Storm Jameson

Preface

We cannot become what we need to be by remaining what we are.

—Max De Pree, businessman and writer.

This is my story about having the nerve to recover from a potentially fatal and life-changing head injury.

There are a few things you need to know about me before we begin. This is not a sob story, and I do not consider myself a victim. Like many, I am a wife, a mother, a sister, and a daughter. However, I'm also a genetics researcher, a physician, and a proud Italian. Some of my earliest memories as a child growing up on Long Island involve the cooking of food, what it represents, and how it ignites the senses. My grandparents were from northern and southern Italy, and our family spoke through the language of food. Meals bring all family members to the table, and we are taught that feeding our family and friends and eating together equals love. You will hear more about my passion with food later on, but maybe it's also important for you to know that I cannot smell anymore. A fragrant basil leaf. A fresh sprig of lavender. While the memories of such smells linger, and I can feign excitement of such normal small pleasures, in reality, my sense of smell is gone. I know I'm cooking onions only because I see them turn translucent, get soft, and I feel the heat of the pan on my face. Unexpected life events alter you and your relationship to the world, and the challenges can be immense.

I graduated from Brown University and University of Cincinnati Medical School, and I trained at Harvard, Mass General Hospital, and the National Institute of Health (NIH). I have two wonderful boys, and my husband, Carlos, is my other half in both work and life. I am fortunate. However, on April 1, 2006, in a split second, everything turned upside down. I nearly lost my head.

At that time, as a new faculty member of the University of Southern California, I was looking forward to my role as Associate Chair of Education in Psychiatry and Director of the Center for Genomic Psychiatry. I was 50 years old, and much of my life seemed set. Carlos and I were moving and shaking in our field as research scientists and doctors. We could, as couples often do, wistfully map our future for 5 years, 10 years, or 20 years.

However, despite all the preparation and hard work, some things, I've learned, are discovered the hard way. How do we account for the toughest type of challenge: an accident and the unknown?

This book presents what happened when a person got hit with the unthinkable. The impossible. The unpredictable. A traumatic brain injury. According to the CDC, more than 1.7 million people in the United States experience traumatic brain injuries (TBIs) every year, with 30% resulting in injury-related deaths. Those who do survive face enormous challenges, requiring a village of rehab therapists, neurosurgeons, and tirelessly supportive family members and friends during and after recovery. As a doctor who has devoted my life's work to the study of the brain and its inner workings, it is somewhat ironic that I suffered a brain injury. In addition, it is unfathomable that, at first, it left me with expressive aphasia, almost a complete inability to speak. In the more than decade and a half that has passed since my injury—a terrible April Fool's joke—I have taken this moment of adversity and turned it into a lesson in resilience.

The scary truth is that TBIs, which can be either mild (concussive, often multiple) or severe (usually a single blow), are becoming increasingly common. If you have ever watched football on TV, you've seen them happen in real time during every game. The health outcomes of TBI survivors vary widely. Aside from the immediate consequences of brain injury (loss of primary functions such as paralysis, inability to eat, and use your five senses), TBIs can also be responsible for early onset dementia, depression, and a host of other cognitive disabilities. However, their prevalence far outpaces the research we are able to conduct. Unlike most diseases that we can replicate and test, in humans, we are only able to study a traumatic brain injury *after* it occurs. For better or worse, depending on how you look at it, each impact and resulting injury is unique. This means that the best practice guidelines for treatment may not apply to every patient; in fact, I guarantee you they don't. Therefore, knowing the patient's abilities and personality before his/her TBI occurred becomes vitally important. Although I will be sharing my personal journey of recovery, I will include tips and expert opinions that can be useful to anyone – a patient, caregiver, and clinician alike—who has a connection to TBI.

Oftentimes with brain injuries, as in my own case of expressive aphasia, the patient is unable to advocate or express what they are thinking and feeling. Therefore, family members and friends become the voice of the patient and must advocate for personalized medical care with professional caregivers. If you are in a recovery phase or struggling with a family member or friend that has TBI, my goal is that you will read this and find new hope and inspiration: Don't be a prisoner of your prognosis. No two patients are the same. Resilience, which is the ability to bounce back, teaches us to never underestimate a person's ability to compensate for their deficits and overcome the odds.

As far as TBIs go, some might say I am a miracle case. However, I would say not so much a miracle as much as I am stubborn and not willing to give up. Maybe I just have a double dose of resilience! Since I survived with the help of so many I wanted to give back. With that, I feel a responsibility to share what I know to be true.

New Brunswick, NJ, USA   Michele T. Pato, MD

Acknowledgments

There are many people to thank for my recovery. I will describe many times the critical and loving role my husband, Carlos, played as my partner for life, perhaps even more important than being a doctor as well.

So many family and friends played important roles at many times and in many different ways.

I must thank my sister, Suzi Tortora, and sister-in-law, Ana Pato Morley. Suzi was at the hospital within hours, and in many ways, this injury was a blessing in disguise, as it has drawn us closer. Ana, living in Syracuse at the time, played a crucial role that made this book possible. She, with the help of her husband, Chris, was instrumental in recording daily notes and keeping all friends and family informed in the initial month of my recovery and beyond. Ana, a talented writer herself, went on to work with me on a draft of the manuscript recounting the first years of my recovery. Her countless hours of interviews, research, and writing helped fill in the gaps in my memory. Ana's contribution of time, effort, and support was fundamental in this endeavor, and I cannot thank her enough. I also must credit my son Eric Tortora Pato for the cover design for the book.

It took working with someone outside of the initial experience to help me to truly understand what was the same and what had changed after my injury. I needed someone with a perspective from the outside looking in, and this is what my editor Rachel Trusheim provided.

Along the way many others have helped. Some I mention by name and others know, without being asked or specifically acknowledged, that they played a role in my recovery. My sons, Michael and Eric, have never stopped helping me in so many ways. Thanks to my Dad and Mom, Tony and Lucille Tortora, who were there from the moment it happened and ever since. Even though Dad is no longer with us, he is still in my daily thoughts, reminding me to move forward. Thanks also to my colleagues and friends: Helena Medieros, Cindy Wojtecki, Cynthia Harrington, James Knowles, Lois Slovik, Barbara Van Noppen, and Mark Rappaport.

While there have been a number of memoirs published, there are rather few written by those with TBI. I want to thank the publisher for taking a chance on me not only as the survivor of TBI but also as a doctor who actually studies the mind and the brain. Thank you for finding this book as unique and revealing as I did.

I hope this memoir provides hope and inspiration to you or a loved one who suffers from TBI. Life is a gift that can be worth living in many different ways. You can't just look back but must always look forward on how to use your gift by living each day.

Contents

.

Grace

1

All things are difficult before they are easy.

—*Thomas Fuller, clergyman*

Even if I knew that tomorrow the world would go to pieces, I would still plant my apple tree.

—*Martin Luther, theologian*

In the first 3 days as I was sedated, placed in medical coma to reduce the rapid swelling in my brain, I am told family and friends from all over came to my bedside. The waiting room was full of Tortoras and Patos, and many more of our close friends and colleagues had journeyed to Pittsburgh from Maryland, New York, and California. My younger sister, Suzi, was called by my father at the scene of the accident, rushed within hours to be with me. It was a call she would never forget, and she dropped everything to come be with me. As a clinical dance/movement therapist, Suzi felt strongly that I needed to be "bathed in music I loved" even while unconscious. She believed that familiar music playing every day in my hospital room was essential for my brain to heal, so Suzi grabbed her iPod and travel speakers with her when she ran to the airport. She loaded it up with music we had grown up with: songs from the 1970s, Carole King hits, and gospel spirituals. The moment she connected the iPod to the speakers in the room, that is when the family started to see some flashes of hope.

Each time the doctors eased back on the amount of sedation in my IV tube, my arms and legs on my left side would tremor and twitch, at times as if I was trying to run in bed. The medical team was so concerned about this that they made multiple efforts to restrain me; however, this was a true sign to Suzi that I was truly inside there and would be okay. It was so like me to be restless and moving my legs all over the place. I wanted to go jogging, as I had every day. Nevertheless, I was not yet conscious, nor was I ever officially upgraded from my "critical" condition. When I

M. T. Pato, *Nerve*, https://doi.org/10.1007/978-3-031-33433-7_1

woke up and heard Suzi's music softly playing in the background, it was not all that surprising that I would move first. I could never sit still in a concert! Although I couldn't do much in those early hours of consciousness, I believe I might have felt the rhythm of the music.

On the evening of April 3, 2006, I was brought out of coma at Allegheny General Hospital in Pittsburgh, 2500 miles from my new home in California. This was the first time I was awake and responsive since what the Commonwealth of Pennsylvania's police crash report called a "motor vehicle versus pedestrian accident" occurred. I woke up with a giant hole in my head.

Suzi played "Amazing Grace" on a daily basis, and she asked to be able to sit with me alone long after everyone had left, which the staff permitted for a short time. She also played music from Carol King's *Welcome to My Living Room* album that I had given her for Christmas. Then, she received permission from the nurses to set up her iPod and speakers to play music for a longer time. Although I had no ability to speak, I was able to sing out a few lines of the hymn "Amazing Grace," with a wide smile spread across my face. In addition, by the time the rest of my family returned to the room, I was also able to join in a sing-along to the music in the background with my mother-in-law, Odette Pato.

The next day when I opened my eyes, I could feel the sunshine warm on my face. As my surroundings pulled into focus, there were people standing around me whom I knew: mom; my sister, Suzi; and my husband, Carlos. I opened my mouth to say, "Hi, I'm okay! Wait…where am I? Why are you here?" However, nothing I was thinking would come out. As a self-described "motor mouth" who almost never let others get two words in edgewise, this was a bizarre feeling.

I could see reflected in my family's faces that I must have made a quizzical frown, wanting to know more. They were cautious and kept their answers simple: "You are in the hospital, Michele. You needed surgery on your head. We are so happy you woke up." Then, Carlos told me, "Three days in coma. They just extubated you." He used the word *extubated*, which we both knew and used routinely as physicians, although in simpler terms it meant only that the doctors had just pulled the breathing tube out of my mouth. Then, he continued, "We're so glad to see you moving and that your eyes are open. We couldn't wake you up." I managed a smile to show him that I understood.

As I lay silent in the all-white room, my family immediately asked me questions: *Do you know where you are? Do you remember what happened? Do you know your name?* I nodded my head and uttered over and over again, "Eric." Everyone was Eric, who was my younger son. My family seemed ecstatic that I was awake. Later, I'd learn how truly terrified they were in this happy moment, alarmed by my errors in speech and memory. Then, Carlos asked once more, "Who am I?" I grinned and tried to answer, "You are *Michele?*" The room erupted in boisterous laughter. After 26 years of marriage, finally, the truth came out. My husband was no longer a separate person!

Having no memory of what had happened or why I was there, I became a bit nervous and started to take in the world around me. I could tell that I was partially sitting up in bed, wearing an itchy hospital gown, and the bed sheet pulled part way up. My throat felt sore and scratchy. With some failed attempts, I realized few words came out of my mouth. I just couldn't make my tongue move well enough to get them out. In my jumbled mind, frustration began to set in. I could hear but not speak my thoughts.

Soon I noticed what was on my head: one of those cheap hockey helmets, made out of Styrofoam and plastic straps, had been hooked under my chin. How was I going to determine what was going on if I couldn't communicate? And now my right arm was barely working, so how could I, with my trademark "doctor's scribble," which began when I was a little girl "learning" penmanship, write anything down?

In one of the rare moments that Carlos allows himself to look back on this life-shattering, tragic time, he recalls that I seemed to smile, not just at the sight of family or occasionally during the day, but *all* of the time. It was as if I never seemed to fully acknowledge or comprehend how horrible and terrifying the injury and subsequent surgery had been. Or maybe I was just happy to be alive.

After days filled with despair, I was able to say, in my own way, that I was going to be okay. Unlike my parents and husband, I had no memory of the 1989 Chevy Blazer careening toward us, or the Buick LeSabre that ran a stop sign and hit the SUV first, or the wrought iron fence my head flew backward into. However, I knew that I was saved. As the song goes, "'Tis Grace has brought me safe thus far and Grace will lead me home."

Head

2

The chief function of the body is to carry the brain around.

—*Thomas A. Edison, inventor*

The human brain has 100 billion neurons, each neuron connected to 10 thousand other neurons. Sitting on your shoulders is the most complicated object in the known universe.

—*Michio Kaku, theoretical physicist*

On October 26, 1956, I was born with a full head of thick black hair to Antonio and Lucille Tortora at Freeport Hospital in Long Island, New York. I grew up in a typical middle-class Italian-American household. I attended Catholic school through the second grade and then transferred to the public school system when my family moved to Merrick, Long Island. The new neighborhood seemed more affluent, the house was bigger, and we had a nicer yard. My mother's younger sister, Anita, and her family eventually moved out to live near us, which was in keeping with our close-knit Italian roots. Therefore, I went to school with my cousins, and family has always played a huge part in my life (Figs. 2.1 and 2.2).

I went through the entire Merrick school district from Old Mill Road Elementary to Brookside Junior High and finally Calhoun High School. It was through those school years that my competitive spirit thrived. My sister, Suzi, was born with natural grace and poise that blossomed into a magnificent talent for dance and gymnastics. I, on the other hand, was far more interested in beating the boys on the soccer field and scoring points. I played soccer, basketball, and volleyball. It was pretty clear at a young age that I was an aggressive player with the drive to push my body to its limits, training rigorously. I pushed my teammates often and loved to win.

At school, I applied myself to every subject, always with an end goal in sight for attaining high honors. Maybe in some ways, my father, an engineer at Grumman Aircraft, rubbed off on me. He inspired me with his groundbreaking work on

M. T. Pato, *Nerve*, https://doi.org/10.1007/978-3-031-33433-7_2

Fig. 2.1 One year old—Eyes wide open and always curious

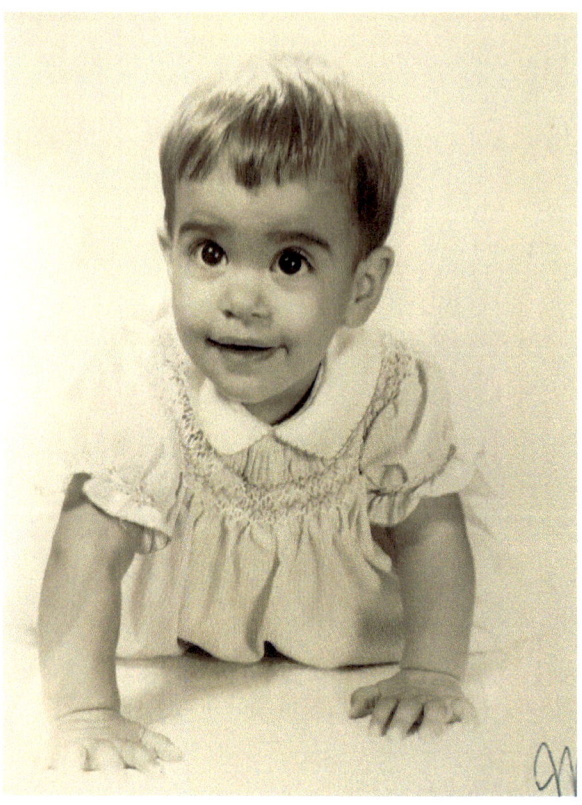

NASA's Mercury, Gemini, Apollo, and Lunar Module. When Apollo 1 exploded shortly after its launch, in addition to being distraught, he was furious and self-critical about what could he do "to fix it" for the next time. Some of my fondest memories are helping with house repairs and learning from him standing side by side, my small frame next to his towering, 6-foot-2-inch 250-pound one. Therefore, it was natural that mathematics and the hard sciences, what we now call STEM, came easiest to me in school. Nevertheless, I wanted to be well rounded, so I also insisted on participating in chorus and orchestra, soccer, yearbook, and the school newspaper. My senior-year AP Calculus teacher, Mrs. Vecchione, absolutely dazzled me. Extremely intelligent, she was one of the few female scientists I had ever met. I spent time with her outside of school and must say the encouragement she showed me made a significant impact on my decision to ultimately pursue a career in science (Fig. 2.3).

In 1974, I graduated high school as valedictorian and was accepted to an Ivy League college. It was a first for a woman in my area to go to Brown University. I was recruited through the still-somewhat-new Title IX initiative (1972) to join Brown's fledgling women's soccer team. As a player there, I was able to witness the goalposts move for women's opportunities. We started out with no uniforms and no dedicated athletic field and were never allowed to play on the men's pitch. However,

Fig. 2.2 Second grade—Looked like mom but scientist like dad

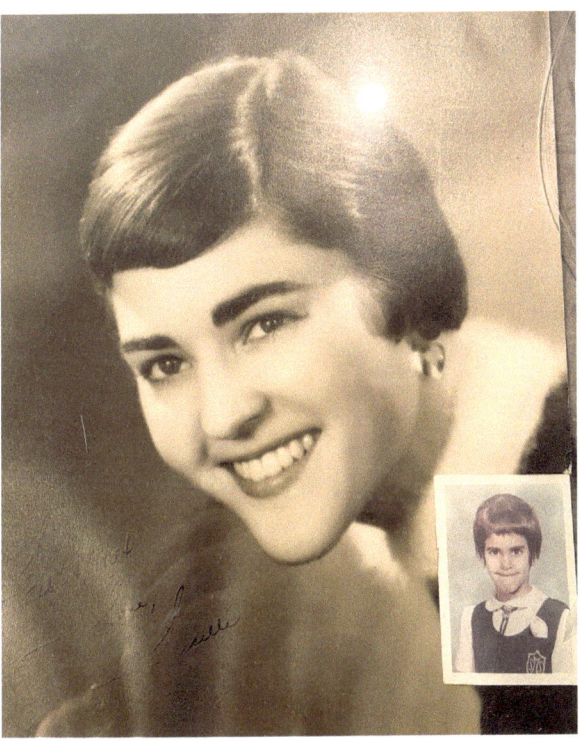

by my last year on the team, we had established ourselves as a respectable contender against other women collegiate soccer teams. We had gained the support of the student body and were rewarded with proper uniforms and practice programs. The personal endurance and athletic stamina that I developed through my soccer training would prove to help save my life, and plenty of experience "heading" the ball probably didn't hurt, either.

It was around that time that Carlos Pato and I first met. It was during our senior year at Brown University in 1977 when he came to visit my suitemate, his girlfriend, at our on-campus apartment. I found him handsome and intriguing. Every time Carlos called our suite, I made sure to answer the phone, eager to hear his voice and say hello before handing the receiver over. When it became apparent in January that they were just friends at this point, I asked my soccer buddy Elaine to tell Carlos I was interested in him, and we went out to dinner within 5 days! In January 1978, after we had been "officially" dating for about week, school was out for winter break, and we found ourselves going to different but nearby ski resorts up in Vermont. One day when rain and ice had closed the slopes, Carlos called me up and asked me to take a road trip with him for lunch. I said, "Sure!" and drove my little car, Audi 100LS, from Sugarbush to Stowe. What I didn't know was that Carlos thought it would be fun to have lunch in Montreal! I had never been out of the country before and didn't have a passport. Luckily, at that time, you could cross the border with a driver's license. It was exhilarating to walk the streets and listen to

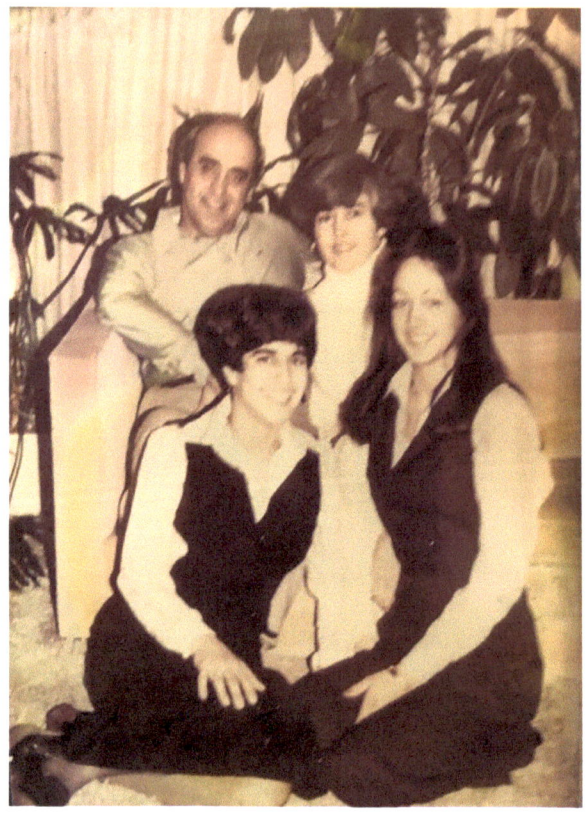

Fig. 2.3 Age 17—Soon to graduate high school as valedictorian and go to Brown University. Typical second generation Italian American family

everyone speak French (a language I had supposedly learned in high school) on a blistery cold day. After lunch, at approximately 4 or 5 p.m., it began snowing. I let Carlos drive, and I became the navigator. We drove in the right lane and I rolled down the window sticking my head out so I could see the edge of the road and to make sure Carlos was heading straight on the highway. Most of the time I was saying, "Go a little left, slightly more left, now go straight." After many hours like this, we finally made it back to Stowe, harrowed but exhilarated. Later in the week, we met up again, and I discovered that Carlos had never skied before! Just as he had taken control of the car in the snowstorm, I took the lead and showed him the ropes while all he could do was hope to be able to stop at the bottom of the slope.

What we learned about each other that week was the basis of the team we are today. I discovered that Carlos could stay the course and was willing to take on new experiences and challenges and that he did not mind me navigating and filling in the details. I could trust in him to make decisions for me and vice versa. All our strengths and complementary skills bonded us then and still do now.

At that time, Carlos was nearing the end of his undergraduate studies, pursuing an 8-year program where he would receive a Bachelor of Arts in Comparative Literature and continue courses in Biochemistry before going to medical school at

Brown. In 1979, I began medical school at the University of Cincinnati, and by July of 1980, we were married. Carlos took a year off so I could catch up and we could be in the same year of medical school. During that year he did research in a bio-chemistry lab in Cincinnati, and then we applied to transfer to each other's medical schools and got in to both. We decided to stay in Cincinnati so Carlos could finish his research where he was most happy and so we could graduate from medical school together. From that point forward, we've been on the same road, different personalities and strengths, but always together in all that we do.

However, on April 1, 2006, while Carlos and I were preparing to cross a street in downtown Pittsburgh, our paths were, for the first time in over a quarter century, dramatically diverted. In a split second, I was struck by a sliding 2-ton SUV. It had been overturned in a T-form collision with a sedan and threw me from the sidewalk into a church's wrought iron fence. I have no memory of the accident, that day, the week prior, or several weeks following, which is called retrograde and antegrade amnesia. Indeed, many of the "memories" from that period that I have recorded here are not so much "recalled" as meticulously rebuilt.

The experience of having to retrace a patch of time within your own life that is lost to you is an incredible journey. It's become a bit of an obsession for me to fill in this huge blank and to understand these events without knowing for sure what is reality and what is my perception. I'm a physician-scientist, so by scouring over medical records and crash investigation reports and by piecing together the accounts of my family and friends who witnessed the accident and its immediate aftermath, this is what I "know" happened.

The spring of 2006 was a chaotic time for Carlos and me. We were coordinating a move across country from Bethesda, Maryland, to Altadena, California, to push forward in our professional careers, which were very much intertwined. We both accepted faculty positions at the University of Southern California in the Department of Psychiatry to build a new approach to large-scale genomic medicine as personal-ized health. That probably sounds like a bunch of jargon, but in essence, our goal was to study how genes and environmental factors play a role in patients' everyday lives. We had just purchased a house in California and were splitting our time between coasts so that our younger son, Eric, could complete his last year of high school in Bethesda, Maryland. He was deep in the college application process and had a few more months left as a senior. Meanwhile, our older son, Michael, was attending Carnegie Mellon University in Pittsburgh as a college sophomore. That same weekend, Carlos's cousin, Susan Neves, an accomplished soprano, was per-forming *Tosca* at the Pittsburgh Opera. Several relatives were making plans to fly in and attend the performance. It was turning into an extended family reunion, and I remember looking immensely forward to the weekend.

The "Strip District," near the Carnegie Mellon campus, oddly felt like home, like any of the Italian neighborhoods I often strolled through. It was full of restaurants, delis, bakeries, and local businesses. A museum was perched at the edge of the neighborhood. It was a busy Saturday morning with the streets full of people buying food for dinner and traffic weaving its way down the narrow streets where some cars had double-parked.

As we stood on the sidewalk in front of Saint Stanislaus Church waiting to cross at the corner of 21st and Smallman streets, it might have occurred to me that it was a strange intersection, maybe more like a parallelogram: the streets not quite meeting at perpendicular angles. To get to the Society of Contemporary Craft museum, we had to use two crosswalks, in other words, to cross the street twice. I was standing in front of this beautiful stone Catholic Church as a part of our group touring the city, which included Carlos, my mother and father, and a friend of a friend, Penny.

Then, a Buick LeSabre, driven by an elderly man in his 80s, was traveling south on 21st Street and failed to stop for the stop sign at the intersection. At that same time, a young man in a Chevrolet Blazer was moving through the intersection, traveling east when the LeSabre collided with it at the rear of the driver side. The impact of the forceful crash flipped the Blazer onto its roof, sliding violently into the sidewalk where it crashed into three pedestrians.

Carlos, Penny, and I were the three pedestrians hit by the overturned SUV. As reported by eyewitnesses, Carlos was thrown airborne for a moment but landed with enough composure to rise quickly to his feet and rush to the others involved in the accident. Penny was also knocked to the ground and injured but in stable condition. Carlos scanned the windows of the upturned vehicle to check for the driver or passengers. The teenage driver was crawling out through the broken back window, past his Boombox speaker, and appeared to be okay. Carlos still had not yet caught sight of me, as I had been leading the group. Several yards away, my head was wedged into the architectural iron fencing of the church. As a physician, Carlos immediately identified my labored gasps of breath as *agonal* or rattled and arrhythmic. Oxygen was not reaching my brain. As I lay on the sidewalk, my eyes were fluttering, and I was unconscious and not responsive. Carlos made a snap decision. Rather than wait for emergency assistance, he pulled my head from between the two fence posts to try and open up my breathing.

I'm told by my mother, Lucille, that she heard a terrible noise, saw Carlos fly into the air before finding me, and then began yelling, "She's dying, get me an ambulance!" My mother, hysterical, fainted on the scene and was attended to by the paramedics. She was then put in a separate ambulance, brought to the same emergency room and treated for her highly anxious and extreme reaction. The first thing that went through her mind was a flashback of when Suzi almost died as a 9-month-old infant from SIDS. My father thankfully resuscitated my baby sister at the time, but when my mother saw *me* in such a state, she must have immediately thought she was going to lose her child all over again. The local Pittsburgh news station, KDKA, reported the accident on TV, and they mistakenly identified my mother as the victim with head trauma, which made the event even more distressing for her.

The City of Pittsburgh EMS Medic 14 team was dispatched at 10:57 a.m. and arrived on the scene within 4 min. The technicians secured my neck with a brace and placed me on a body board to protect the rest of my spine. Then, as Carlos identified himself as a doctor, they followed his instructions to take me to the hospital immediately, to "scoop and run" rather than "stay and play." After I slid inside the ambulance, Carlos was allowed to ride along in the front seat, probably more because he was a doctor and not because he was my husband. Sirens wailed as we made our way to the hospital. While I was being examined in the ambulance, I vomited blood, which helped to clear my airway. Although I don't remember anything I said or did before or after the accident, the EMS report suggests that I regained consciousness. In fact, I kept trying to pull my oxygen mask off and insisted to the crew that I needed to talk and sit up.

During the short ride, Carlos called a colleague at the University of Pittsburgh to make sure that we were going to the best hospital for head trauma. The EMT protocol directs the ambulance to the nearest hospital, and we learned from a traumatic snowboarding accident involving our son, Michael, that not every hospital is equipped to handle special cases. Our friend confirmed that Allegheny General's head trauma unit was the best one around. The neurosurgeon on call in the emergency room was the very surgeon involved in a historic rescue of miners who were trapped in coal mines in Pennsylvania. This brought comfort to my family: they thought he was the perfect doctor who had extensive experience in severe head injuries.

Meanwhile, 400 miles away in Syracuse, Carlos's sister, Ana, received a telephone call from their mother, Odette, who had been a neonatal nurse. Odette had been summoned from the hotel she was staying at in Pittsburgh to attend the opera performance and was en route to the hospital to be with Carlos. Her voice possessed the eerie, atonal quality of a woman in shock when she spoke the words, "Listen, Ana, there has been an accident. Carlos and Michele have been hurt. It is very serious for Michele. We need to tell the boys to take a taxi to the hospital, RIGHT NOW. I don't have their phone numbers. I don't know anything else." Ana's mind raced with questions she knew her mother had no answers for in her present state. She then hung up to break the hideous news to Michael and Eric about what had happened.

At 11:24 a.m., we arrived at Allegheny General. Carlos sat alone on a bed curtained-off from the rest of the emergency ward, waiting for his own patient assessment to take place. Frustrated and unconcerned with his well-being, he hopped up, declined treatment, and set out to find me in the corridors of the emergency wing while limping. When Carlos located the neurosurgical trauma team, he was shown my CAT scans. Examining them with the neurosurgeon, he zeroed in on the gravity of my injuries. He could see a skull fracture, multiple bleeds, and a midline shift of the brain, indicative of mounting pressure. The two hemispheres of the brain typically look almost like mirror images of each other. However, mine did not; swelling was pushing the left side of my brain into the right.

If the pressure within my skull continued to build up with nowhere to go, it would continue down into the brainstem, which is connected to the top of my spinal cord, risking almost certain death from herniation (swelling of the brain and the pressure on the brainstem against the bony opening at the bottom of the skull, the foramen magnum). Carlos already knew that I urgently needed surgery to release the pressure that was dangerously building. Typically, for traumatic brain injuries, a neurosurgeon will drill what are called burr holes into the skull and give medications to decrease swelling. A more dramatic option, a hemicraniectomy, removes an entire portion of the skull. Practice guidelines, established back in 1979*, consider this to be an extreme if not somewhat barbaric procedure, with a long recovery ahead. Once part of the skull is removed and the edema (swelling) subsides, the patient then waits 3–6 months before cranioplasty, the procedure to restore the intact skull or, in my case, placing my own bone back. Whatever decision was made in those fraught moments would determine the course of our lives.

The neurosurgeon was eager to intervene since it was so soon after a traumatic head injury. He and Carlos agreed, given the amount of swelling in such a short period of time (30 min), the hemicraniectomy would give me the best chance to survive. Had Carlos waited at the scene, allowing the swelling to get even worse, things may have been very different.

My thick hair was hastily shorn off, leaving my head bald for the first time in my life, and the cutting began.

Brain or Bone?

3

To achieve great things, two things are needed: a plan, and not quite enough time.

—Leonard Bernstein

I am not what happened to me, I am what I choose to become.

—Carl Jung, psychiatrist

According to the Centers for Disease Control (CDC), there are 130.4 million emergency room visits in America's hospitals every year. Americans undergo an average of 9.2 surgical procedures in their lifetime. * So it's likely that most everyone will, at one point in their lives, experience some sort of surgery, visit an operating or emergency room, and possibly be put under general anesthesia. As both a physician and a mother who has seen more than a medical ordeal or two, I can attest that it's a harrowing experience to watch on the sidelines. After prolonged periods of waiting, when patients and family members do get to see the doctor, they are hit with a barrage of medical terms they've probably never heard of before and which are difficult to comprehend. In my case of traumatic brain injury (TBI), I have no memory of it whatsoever. As a research psychiatrist specializing in OCD and driven by raw data, this fact drives me nuts, even to this day.

I am uniquely fortunate, however, to be in possession of detailed hospital medical records from my accident, surgeries, and recovery. Medical reports, orders for treatment, and other such forms are not often shared with patients and for good reason. They can be impossible to understand, and as the Hippocratic Oath demands, we as doctors must "first do no harm" to our patients. Sometimes too much information, unfiltered and unwieldy, overwhelms and disturbs the patient even more. However, for me, a person who has no memory of the procedure or how I got to Allegheny General that day, these records have become vital to my understanding of those events and how it could be possible that I am alive to tell the tale. The use

M. T. Pato, *Nerve*, https://doi.org/10.1007/978-3-031-33433-7_3

of medical terms around me, even when they weren't sure I completely understood, seemed to help me retrieve things I knew. This made me feel that I was being treated as the person I was, and not as a patient who wouldn't understand what was being said to me.

Throughout this account, I am choosing to include verbatim excerpts from my records. Where possible, I attempt to provide definitions and lay explanations. There is also a selected glossary of medical terms at the end as well.

The "Indications" section of the hospital's medical report for April 1, 2006 reads Fig. 3.1:

> This 49-year-old woman was injured in a pedestrian versus motor vehicle accident this afternoon.
>
> She was brought to the Allegheny General Hospital Emergency Department, and a trauma alert was called. The trauma service evaluated the patient and called the neurosurgical service. A CT scan of the head revealed an acute left-sided subdural hematoma with 9 mm of brain shift at the midline, out of proportion to the size of the subdural hematoma (blood clot). We discussed the situation with her husband and recommended a decompressive hemicraniectomy for presumed postaccident swelling. The risks and benefits of the procedure were explained to him, and he wished to proceed.

In hindsight, I have no doubt that when Carlos signed off on the operative procedure above called a "left decompressive hemicraniectomy," he must have thought, *Dear God, the most important thing to Michele is her brain*. To relieve pressure from a swelling brain tissue and "evacuate the subdural hematoma" both contributing to the brain shift from midline and which had formed after impact, neurosurgeons would remove half of my skull bone from the top of my head, spanning directly above my left eye to my left ear. Even in modern times, removing such a

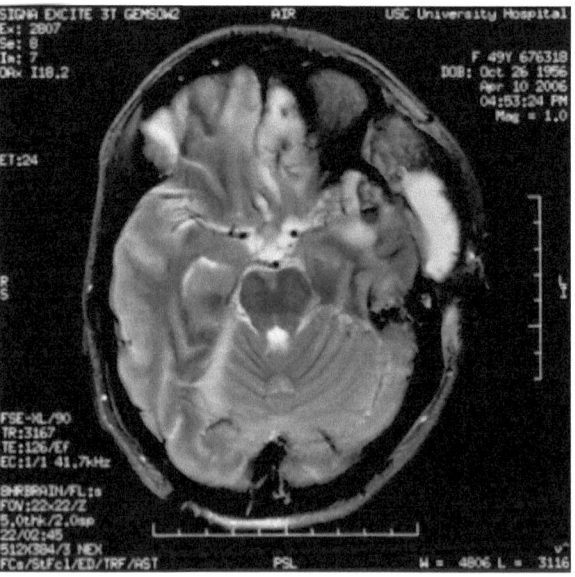

Fig. 3.1 My MRI—Day 10—the blood clot (subdural hematoma) on my left brain above my left ear

large section of skull seems extreme and barbaric. As the report states, Carlos was informed of the risks. As a husband and a physician, he had to make a life-changing decision for both of us. We were each other's yin and yang. Left and right. Two parts of a whole. I know in that moment Carlos must have felt rudderless. A plane that had lost a wing and was barreling lopsided toward the ground.

Single, severe TBI (ssTBI) can be particularly cruel to both the patient and their loved ones. The result of a fall, blow, or crash and subsequent impact, a perfectly healthy brain, now injured, fights against its own skull as it swells. In many cases of TBI, survival is the best outcome, with no consideration for quality of life or regaining cognitive functions. In many cases, given the severity of TBI, survival alone is the goal. The surgeon might argue that survival is the only reasonable outcome. This may well be true, since recovery is so unique to each individual and so unpredictable. After all, ssTBI is not a condition that can be freely studied in larger data sets from willing participants in a controlled environment. As a survivor who struggled and succeeded with recovery despite my terrible prognosis, I'm glad they offered to do the risky surgery and that Carlos said yes. However, I wonder about others. Are there better ways of predicting the prognosis, quality of life, or cognitive functions one might regain? Perhaps this is part of my motivation in writing this book. By understanding resilience and conducting more research in this area, we could better predict and guide recovery.

A hemicraniectomy would remove a large section of bone to save the brain, but there was no guarantee that the operation would be successful at stopping the swelling, that the surgeons would not damage the brain while performing it, or that I would recover at all.

With my fate sealed, so to speak, the surgeons carefully proceeded; as I lay supine on the operating table, my scalp prepped in a sterile fashion:

> A large [skin] flap was planned, extending from the frontal hairline to the transverse sinus. Incision was made with a 10 blade knife down to the subcutaneous fat. Meticulous hemostasis was achieved with monopolar cautery. With the help of monopolar cautery, we turned a musculocutaneous flap with a minimal amount of blood loss. Four burr holes were made at the frontal, parietal and temporal bone with the high-speed drill. The craniotomy was used to complete the [bone] flap. The dura [mater] was taut and evidently under quite a bit of pressure. We opened the dura and allowed the brain to relax. Copious amounts of hematoma were evacuated from beneath the dura. We continued to evacuate the hematoma with copious amounts of saline and suction. The frontal and temporal lobes were contused [bruised], and we made sure to check for any occult [unseen] bleeding. The vein which may represent the Labbe was adherent to the dura. For this reason, we cut the dura out so as to release the vein from tension. We would recommend that future surgeons working in this area be careful of avulsing this vein.

More simply put, the surgeons mapped and then cut out a large section of my left skull before penetrating the brain to locate and suck out the pool of blood (subdural hematoma from torn arteries and veins) that had been caused by the injury. In between the skull and brain are membranes called the meninges, which contain three layers of tissue: the dura, arachnoid, and pia mater. See the illustration* below

for an example of a subdural hematoma versus a normal, uninjured brain: https://
www.thoughtco.com/brain-anatomy-meninges-4018883

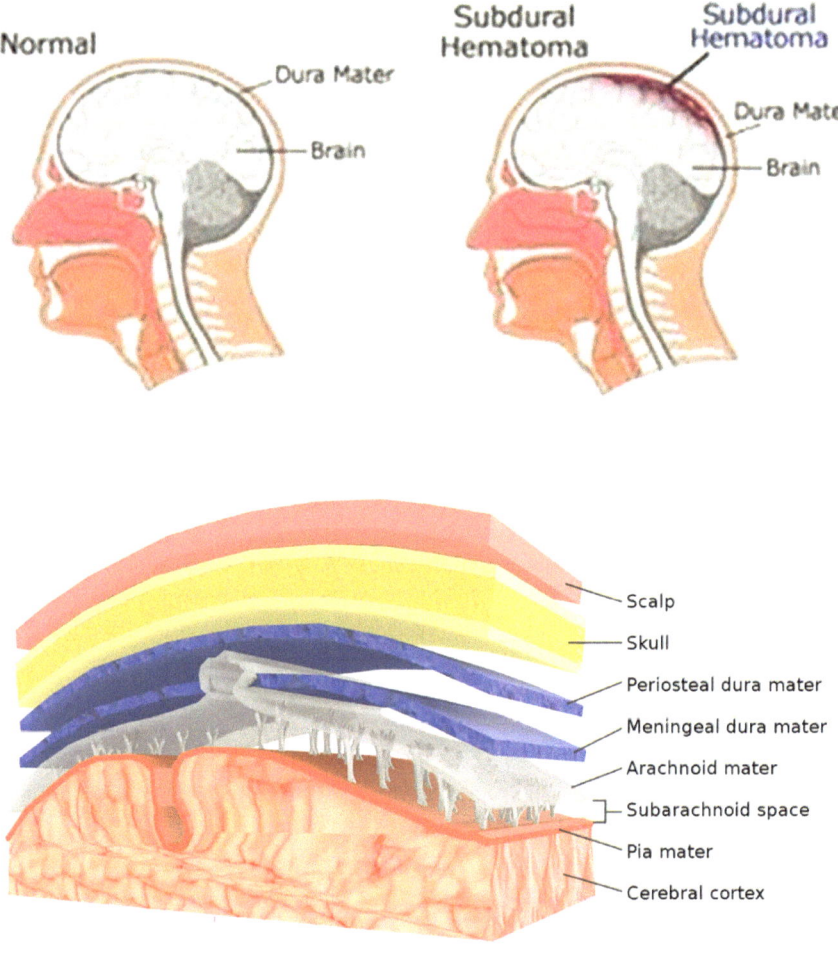

Used with permission, Evelyn Bailey.

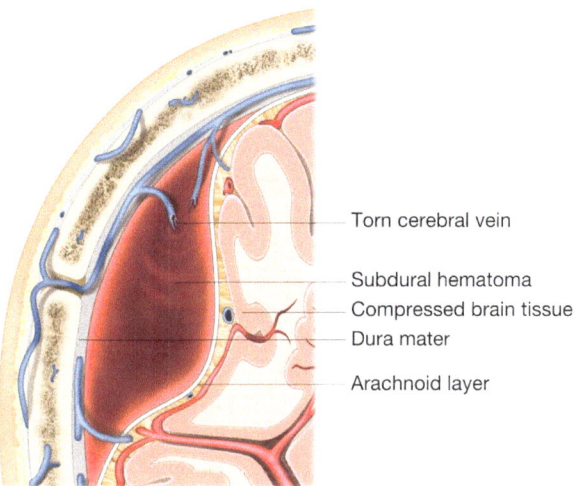

Torn cerebral vein

Subdural hematoma
Compressed brain tissue
Dura mater

Arachnoid layer

Once they were able to stop the bleeding by cauterizing the surrounding veins, there was the matter of stabilizing the brain without replacing the bone. To do so, they had to place Gelfilm, similar to an artificial layer of meninges, over the exposed brain layers to allow healing. Then, they had to flap my scalp back over and stitch me up:

> After meticulous hemostasis [stopping the bleeding] was achieved, we placed Gelfilm over the dura, which had been opened in numerous areas to allow the brain to fully relax. Two 10 black drains were left underneath the skin flap to prevent postoperative hematoma recurrence. The flap was closed with interrupted 2-0 Polysorb subgaleal stitches. The skin was closed tightly with staples, and the wound was washed, dried and dressed sterilely. The patient was awakened from anesthesia and transferred to the trauma intensive care unit.

To give some perspective on the scale of the surgery, I received 150 stitches to close the incision, which was 8–9 inches long. With that large amount of bone missing, the report fails to specify where in the world it went or what would happen to it. Typically, a removed bone plate is stored within the body (yes, you read this correctly!) under the omentum, a double layer of fatty tissue that covers and supports the intestines and organs in the lower abdominal area. This is done to keep the bone alive, and there is no better host for a bone than its own environment. However, when I was struck by the overturned Chevy Blazer and thrown into the iron fence, I also sustained internal injuries in the form of lacerations to my liver and right kidney. The surgeons did not want to open my abdomen while I was still bleeding from my liver and kidney, fearing more trauma and blood loss. This meant that the bone had to be placed in deep freeze storage, which is less than ideal but was necessary if there was any hope of putting back my own bone and not some synthetic substitute back.

Why share this information? In addition to identifying a huge gap in my own memory, I hope to shed some light on what TBI patients experience and need to recover from. However, common TBIs are almost always unexpected. Families are faced with life and death decisions to make while being introduced to a crash course in neuroscience and traumatic brain injury. Although the procedure in many ways is violent, I have no doubt that the decision to remove part of my skull was the right call for me. There were a few lucky breaks in all of this that I believe went my way, and although I credit my recovery to a multitude of things, I have to believe that somewhere the odds were slightly in my favor.

During the operation and later, as I remained sedated in a medically induced coma, I am told that Carlos, in the waiting room with upward of 20 close family members and friends, spoke of all we had been through in our life together. He reflected on all the difficult moments, times when we had taken each other for granted, and how devastating the prospect of losing me, his wife of 25 years and mother to his children, would be. Carlos is always solution focused, so in the immediate period, he would be constantly evaluating next steps and how to "solve" the problem. At this time, it was premature to lose hope, and each moment he was focused on the next.

My sister, Suzi, took it upon herself to see that everyone was cared for as best as possible. She comforted our overwrought mother and tried to assist her with relaxation techniques. She listened carefully to our father's concerns and worries and took notes, at times, to find answers to his questions when possible. She listened attentively to every piece of information that Carlos and the attending medical team had to offer. It was clear to her that Carlos was walking more and more with a pronounced limp but refusing to receive care for his own injuries.

In similar situations in the past, I would have been the one to interpret the facts and offer a deeper insight from a medical perspective to the family of a loved one. I was counted upon to pinpoint the "positives" in the vital statistics and offer a little peace during a tough time. I would have fielded questions when there was a nagging concern. My family had no such counsel as they waited for me to wake up. Carlos was consumed with making medical decisions and focused on me and our children's needs, and Ana, Carlos's sister who was back in Syracuse, did her best to learn everything about traumatic brain injury that she could on the Internet, but there was still an empty space where my opinions, support, and laughter usually lingered.

Now I just had to wake up.

Nerves

4

Follow your heart but take your brain with you.

—Alfred Adler, psychotherapist

Each day is a little life: every waking and rising a little birth,
every fresh morning a little youth, every going to rest and sleep
a little death.

—Arthur Schopenhauer, philosopher

After the surgery, I was wheeled over to the intensive care unit in critical condition. That evening, friends and family, who had flown in to see Carlos's cousin, Susan Neves, perform at the opera, resolved to go and show their support. My sister, Suzi, stayed behind with me, and Carlos and Eric went to the show but left at intermission. Before the performance, Susan made a special announcement asking the audience to keep me in their prayers.

Afterward, most of my family retreated to the hotel under great strain. After seeing to it that our parents were resting in their hotel room, Suzi went to check in on Carlos. Neither could sleep. Carlos was on the phone with the hospital throughout the night to keep apprised of any change to my condition. She found him in a high state of both vigilance and exhaustion. Suzi tried to convince Carlos to admit that his limp was obvious, and she pointed out that he was not moving one of his knees in a normal way. The recognition of the injury snapped Carlos out of the adrenaline-fueled state he'd been in since the crisis began that morning. The realities were beginning to sink in. He seemed to not register that he was a victim of the accident as well.

That night, Suzi asked Carlos if he would like her to sit with him for a while in his room. She told him she was trained in a massage technique called "connective tissue massage" and that if used on his knee, it would help to lower the swelling and feel better. He agreed. He sat up on his bed with his leg elevated with a pillow, and

Suzi sat at the end of the bed holding his knee and leg in her hands. Connective tissue massage is a very gentle technique that uses the side of your fingers to lift the fascia. It can feel like a sharp line under your skin at the place of contact and can also create sensations in other areas of the body not related at all to the site of contact. In this way, it creates an overall relaxation state. In a few minutes, she began to talk with Carlos, just asking him to tell her about what was on his mind and what he and I were up to regarding our new jobs and move to the West Coast. Carlos began to talk and slowly opened up about our life together over all the years that we had known each other. They talked the whole night into the morning. He spoke about our relationship, how he felt when he first met me, and explored past family dynamics. Suzi decided to encourage him to speak, feeling that the more he reminisced, the more alive I was in his mind. It led Carlos to tell Suzi, "Now I know why you are such a good therapist!"

At one point, he commented that even though they had been brother- and sister-in-law for so many years, they had never truly spoken in such depth before, which was true. He expressed regrets, and Suzi decided in that moment to let the past go. Especially in times of crisis, there can be opportunities to bond and grow.

The next day, while I was sedated and the medication began to wear off, I would open my eyes and respond to verbal commands from doctors and nurses, such as a hand squeeze or a finger raise. I also displayed some mild right-side paresis (muscle weakness); however, my cardiovascular status was excellent, perhaps due to my daily habit of running since the age of 17. The neurosurgeons believed that I might survive, but the risk of infection was high. My initial recovery was estimated at about a year, if all went *perfectly* according to plan.

The neurosurgeons and nurses told Suzi that I was an "antsy" and active person/patient and required more sedation than they had anticipated. I'm sure inherent nerve, or nerviness, was apparent even just moments after I was injured. The EMS report remarks that on the scene of the accident and during the ride in the ambulance, I was agitated and somewhat combative. During my medical coma, each day there was a standing order that I be kept in physical restraints so that I would not pull out my breathing tube or IV. This is because in some cases, disoriented patients become agitated and try to remove the tubes. Nevertheless, to be blunt, as I so often am, this physical activity is not what you'd expect from someone with a head injury of such extreme magnitude. If I had hit the fence an inch to the left or right, I might have become a vegetable. Thankfully, such an outcome was inconceivable to me.

My family tells me that I found ways to communicate and be like myself just hours after waking from my coma on April 3rd. Nevertheless, my cognitive abilities were unknown. I was able, through smiling and recognizing loved ones, to express my joy that I was alive. Compensating for my aphasia, I found amusing ways to respond to inquiries. Carlos asked that evening if I knew where I was, I was able to answer affirmatively. When he told me I needed to get some rest and that he would be back at 8:00 p.m. When visiting hours resumed, I was able to tell him to *not* come back! Because I needed rest! This response was totally true to my character. Initially, calling everyone by my younger son's name, Eric, was touching to him and funny to others; however, my family became concerned about what it might suggest about my long-term injuries. Any expectation that I could have woken up with all of my faculties intact after such an injury and surgery was an absolutely unrealistic notion, but it was not unrealistic to me or my personality.

Now that I was breathing on my own and responding appropriately to stimuli, the doctors began to focus on an assessment and rehabilitation plan for future care. No one quite knew how long I would need to stay hospitalized. Again, remembering every case is unique. There are no "controlled trials" for ssTBI. This can be especially frustrating to loved ones and patients who want clear answers and realistic expectations. I can imagine that the conversations between my healthcare providers and loved ones became so fluid that it's difficult to piece together what was said and by whom. Ana, my sister-in-law, recalls that it was never easy to know which emotion to assign to the latest details they learned. Oftentimes, the prognoses felt less than encouraging to them, peppered with cautionary phrases such as "that is, if she survives the next days or weeks or months without suffering a stroke, or a brain hemorrhage," and "Even then we cannot be sure what her functioning will be like." Unable to properly express myself, it was challenging for those around me to gauge what skills I might or might not regain, and they speculated on "possible disabilities" and "permanent deficits."

The most ominous prediction came just 1 week after the accident, when Carlos was advised by the neurosurgeon that my cognitive skills might never exceed past the mental age of 8. Worse still, no one had the slightest inkling of what I knew of this fate. Looking back on this fuzzy time, I wonder if I had blind faith and determination that I would overcome the injury, or if I was just aiming at surpassing rehab goals so that I could leave the hospital. Suzi recalls that as soon as I could communicate to some degree, I expressed my desire to get back to running as soon as possible, and it was unacceptable to contemplate never jogging again. Convalescing has never been my thing! I have to believe that I never lost faith that I would meet the next challenge in front of me. It reminds me that patients in coma or left without the ability to express themselves, as I couldn't, may well have a better understanding of their surroundings than you may think.

This whole process was extremely exhausting for Carlos and my sons, Michael and Eric. Carlos, vacillating between husband and doctor, had avoided looking at the future by grounding himself almost completely to the present. I'm told that he divided his time between managing my medical care and attending to the other necessary aspects of our lives and his new job as Chair of Psychiatry and delegated whenever possible. Carlos was consumed with minute-to-minute, black-and-white decisions. Once he heard that bleak prognosis, it became a reality that if I did survive, my life might be challenged with permanent physical, cognitive, or behavioral impairments. This was the first time that Carlos questioned the decision to treat aggressively. He wondered if I would have wanted to live if I was seriously compromised.

My recovery, at least to those around me, with a guarded prognosis from the medical caregivers, had no foreseeable finish line. Even if rehabilitation and therapy could reteach all I needed to relearn, complications could riddle me for the rest of my days. Although it was beyond miraculous that I had survived (which is all one can hope for, right?), now there was the burden of recovery to face. I'm sure this caused Carlos to be wracked with worry and guilt. Had he made the wrong decision? Would I ever be Michele again?

Not long before the accident, Carlos and I had had a frank discussion about mortality. We made an outline of plans for a future if one of us were to die. Neither of us wanted extraordinary measures to keep us alive if we could not function. In addition, when it came to disability, especially one affecting our ability to function cognitively and emotionally, we loved each other enough to want the other to continue on in life and work. This meant that we would provide the very best care for each other while giving permission for the caretaker to be "free" and carry on.

However, there I was, struggling from within to get out. In the early days, there were some remarkable moments of progress. I was able smile at my sister-in-law and call her "Ana" on the first try. I could carry on short, guided conversations with my parents, hug cousins, and giggle for friends. Parts of my personality began to show as soon as April 5th: I blew my family a kiss, I greeted a friend with my trademark "Hey, you!" and I ambled a few steps with the help of two nurses. Even though my right side was still somewhat paralyzed, my nerves were showing I was ready to take on the next challenge. So much so, I wanted to get the heck out of Pittsburgh!

Mind

5

> *You have power over your mind – not outside events. Realize this, and you will find strength.*
>
> —Marcus Aurelius, Roman emperor (121–180 AD)

As the days passed in Allegheny General, it was becoming clear that my subsequent cranioplasty—the operation to put the part of my skull back—and other practical aspects of my recovery would need to take place somewhere else. The only thing I could express clearly at the time was my wish for an early discharge from the hospital. There's an old Italian credo that you only need to be in the hospital if you are dying!

Therefore, on the morning of April seventh, after some improvement with my internal injuries and reduced swelling in my brain, I was flown by MedEvac plane to Los Angeles. A dear colleague, C.L. Max Nikias, the provost of USC at that time, had generously arranged for the flight along with my insurance so I could be treated close to my new home. The cross-country trip was scheduled to make one pit stop in Nevada before arriving at LAX. Then, I was to continue my care in the ICU at USC University Hospital. The small jet aircraft carried two pilots, two medical professionals (a nurse and a paramedic), and Carlos (physician and husband), along with all the emergency life-support equipment necessary (defibrillator, ventilator, heart monitor, among other things), should something go wrong. It was literally an ambulance in the air. I was placed on a stretcher, strapped tightly to avoid jostling during the flight, and outfitted with the now-dreaded protective helmet. Over the course of the 5-hour flight, I'm told I was quite friendly with the crew and had Carlos's help translating my story to them. Then, just as the pilot began to descend into the City of Los Angeles, I caught a glimpse out the window of a California mountain range like the one near my new home in Altadena. I asked the pilots to just drop me off if it was not too out of the way. Everyone on the plane laughed, but there's a kernel of truth within every joke. I truly thought I could already go home.

M. T. Pato, *Nerve*, https://doi.org/10.1007/978-3-031-33433-7_5

I just couldn't accept I was not yet recovered enough. Was this lack of insight, brain damage, determination, stubbornness, or just my own built-in resiliency? Maybe all of the above? It's hard to say. You choose!

In the time leading up to and including my transfer to USC, I am told that I forcefully asserted that I was "feeling better" but often failed to recognize people, remember facts, or use correct words for the objects around me. According to Ana, I was incredulous over the need to be in a hospital at all! Coupled with a combative (or, as I prefer, determined) nature that was previously evident from the EMS accident report, I seemed to disagree with others about the nature of my true condition. When Carlos corrected my words or actions, such as treating a visiting friend as a nurse or calling the saltshaker a "key," it was beyond difficult to accept. Given the injuries to my left temporal and bilateral frontal lobes, I'm not sure I was aware that my expressive aphasia caused me to use the wrong words. Having no working memory of the accident made it suddenly feel as though Carlos was treating me unkindly for no reason. Later, it became clear that these were symptoms of the brain injury, but my loved ones still had to cope with dramatic changes in my personality and behavior.

Any struggles between Carlos and me during this time would not be considered unique in cases of TBI. Often, the first behavioral challenge TBI patients and their family face is that brain injuries can diminish self-awareness. This is especially true with head injuries that strike the frontal lobe of the brain, which regulates executive functioning. Although I believe I felt like myself inside, my behaviors and speech were betraying my mind. Carlos benefitted from his expertise and understanding of these behavioral manifestations of my injury. This helped him deal with my blaming him for being in the hospital. For many families, without our unique background, this can be especially hard.

While in retrospect I greatly sympathize with my friends and family, at the time I remember being both extremely hopeful that I would recover and frustrated that it was not happening quickly enough. Rehabilitation physician Kathleen Bell, MD, warns that relatives often take it on the chin. Such professionals will recommend that it is wise to curtail conversations with TBI patients who may lead to misunderstandings. The need to avoid problematic topics becomes as crucial as every other aspect of their care. However, in the era of personalized medicine, it may also be necessary to know what the patient would most benefit from. Keeping the TBI patient engaged in positive topics and activities is beneficial for stabilizing mood. In my case, the mere suggestion of doing something other than "Michele's way" could lead to intense moodiness. As I progressed in rehab, I wanted to go home and felt that Carlos should be able to convince the doctors. If I wasn't discharged immediately, it was because Carlos was punishing me. I told him that if he could not take me home, he shouldn't bother visiting. Again, Carlos's expertise helped him understand what was happening and not take any of this personally. At the same time, if I did not have everything explained to me in complex medical terms would have made me feel infantilized.

Many of my friends and family members understood that my contrary attitude was temporary, but Carlos gently and consistently pushed back. This made me even more angry. However, I knew that when he expected me to act reasonably, he was respecting my agency as an adult rather than treating me like a child. I'm told Carlos tried to avoid letting the medical and behavioral interventions I needed compromise my autonomy any more than necessary. After a while I realized that what Carlos wanted me to do was what I was capable of. It started to feel like others were counting me out, but Carlos wasn't going to let it go down that way. When I look back, it was Carlos and my children who gave me back enough of myself to get through the whole ordeal.

Michael and Eric, who were both young adults at the time, were aware of the severity of the situation, yet they possessed different outlooks. Michael, who was completing his sophomore year at Carnegie Mellon University at the time of the accident, said it was clear to him there would be long-lasting effects, which I'm sure created a sense of guilt for him. Over time, he took his father's lead on what to expect more from me and did so with great tenderness. That didn't prevent him from offering anything he could to assist his me in my recovery, even a blood transfusion or one of his kidneys, if needed. Michael made frequent visits the 7 days I was in Pittsburgh and stayed connected to me daily, even from a distance when I moved to California for the rest of my recovery period.

Michael did not come to California but stayed in school in Pittsburgh. I think in part because he knew it was what Carlos and I wanted. Over the years, Carlos and I moved seven or eight times around the country as we took various academic positions, but a priority in every move was making sure it would not interfere with our kids' schooling. Michael was excelling in his second year at Carnegie Mellon, and as parents, we would not want anything, even my accident, to disrupt that.

This was not Michael's first experience with coping with a medical challenge either, and perhaps that is why he could still be hopeful and willing to help. At age 14, he was an avid snowboarder. During one run, he quickly turned to avoid hitting a novice skier who had fallen in front of him, straight into a huge tree he'd missed in his peripheral vision. Although he was wearing a helmet, he crushed his face and needed over 300 stitches as well as ocular and facial reconstruction. He wore an eye patch and had to refrain from activities that required eye movement. It's pretty hard not to move your eyes conjointly when we are naturally programmed for that from birth. Therefore, the best way to help his left eye heal was not to move his right eye much either. I stayed home with him for several weeks, reading books to him and listening to music while his bones healed. However, Michael insisted on snowboarding the first day of the season the next winter in Buffalo (Fig. 5.1).

My younger child, Eric, was in a different place in his life as a high school senior in Bethesda, Maryland (Fig. 5.1). When the accident happened, he remained resolute that I, his mother, would never give up, no matter what the future held. However, it had an enormous impact on Eric's life. At that time, Eric was living in Bethesda, Maryland, with me, where the plan had been to see him through graduation before I would move out more permanently to the West Coast to be with Carlos. Carlos had already begun his job at USC on New Year's Day 2016. While he was tackling the relocation of the infrastructure for our current research project, there was also a big life decision for Eric to make about which college he would attend. Eric was

Fig. 5.1 Eric and Michele
in Pittsburgh I.C.U. on day
6 after awakening
from Coma

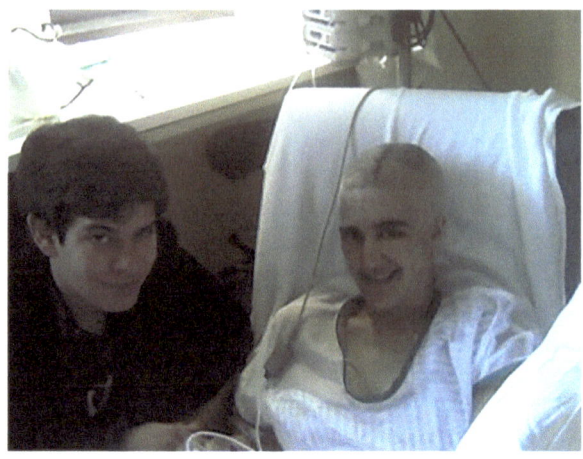

undergoing the college application/acceptance process, and it was April, so he still
had 2–3 months before he was to graduate. In the wake of the events, Eric made a
very adult decision to stay by my side. This is the letter he sent off to his high school
principal:

> From: Eric Pato
> Date: Sun, Apr 2, 2006 at 4:25 AM
> Subject: An Important Note
> Dear Mr. Burgess,
> I am sending out a letter to all of my teachers explaining that for the next week, April
> 3rd to the 7th, I will unfortunately not be attending any of my classes. Please believe me
> when I say I would vastly prefer to be in class and participating, but due to certain events I
> have had to change my priorities. This is because earlier today, my parents were involved in
> a traffic accident while we were visiting my brother in Pittsburgh where a van that was
> struck and flipped on its roof slid into the sidewalk, colliding with them and a friend of the
> family. Although our friend is fine and my father miraculously had only bruising, my
> mother was not as lucky. She suffered serious head trauma and had to go in for brain surgery
> today, and although she is stable now, it will take several days for us to know anything for
> sure or for her to even regain consciousness. As such, I decided I need to be here.
> I will try to stay up to date in classes by getting information from my friends in the
> respective courses, but it is not likely I will be fully up to date. I hope to return to all your
> classes on Monday the 17th with good news. Thank you in advance for your understanding
> and your support.
>
> —Eric Pato

It occurs to me that while I felt misunderstood during much of this critical time,
those nearest to me showed unwavering support. Although I wasn't yet of sound
body, they always believed that I would return to a sound mind.

Eric never returned to classes with the rest of his classmates. The school made
arrangements with Carlos to permit him to finish his senior year by correspondence.
He did not attend award ceremonies or participate in senior traditions that usually
mark a graduate's late spring semester. However, he submitted every assignment,
completed his requirements, and graduated on time. In addition, he had to decide

where to attend college. This was an important decision between two of his top schools: USC, where Carlos and I were now on faculty and could offer him a "free ride," or NYU's Film Program at the Tisch School of the Arts. There might have been some pressure on him to enroll at USC, but we encouraged him to go where he would be happiest, and that was to pursue film at NYU. Eric returned to Maryland in June to participate in his graduation ceremony. The best moment, as Eric reported on that day, was that his mother was able to board a plane and travel to be with him.

Impatient Patient

6

The two most powerful warriors are patience and time.

—*Leo Tolstoy, author*

Patience and perseverance have a magical effect before which difficulties disappear and obstacles vanish.

—*John Quincy Adams, US president*

I have just three things to teach: simplicity, patience, compassion. These three are your greatest treasures.

—*Lao Tzu, philosopher*

Upon admittance at USC University Hospital, on April seventh, the doctor noted in my medical file: "The patient is awake and alert. She is oriented to her name and place. Her speech is fluent, though at times nonsensical. She is able to name objects such as a pen and watch." I spent a total of 7 days in USC University Hospital undergoing tests, physical therapy, and occupational therapy before being relocated to Cedars-Sinai Medical Center's Peters Rehabilitation Hospital for further rehabilitation on Thursday the 13th. The day before I was moved, Michael, by phone with Carlos, expressed some curiosity about how far my language skills had progressed. Carlos decided to test me by asking if I remembered any Portuguese, which I had learned in college after we started dating, because his family is from Portugal. I proclaimed, "Estou pronta para ir para casa!", which means, "I am ready to go home!"

I wish I could say that I was the perfect patient, but my family might seriously disagree. Although I was making great progress in therapy, my requests to go home were dogged and frequent. Carlos felt I was holding him responsible for not being discharged. I even threatened not to talk to anyone unless I was at home. When I was pressed to explain why, I told them I wanted to return to work and tackle a to-do list

© The Author(s), under exclusive license to Springer Nature Switzerland AG 2023   29
M. T. Pato, *Nerve*, https://doi.org/10.1007/978-3-031-33433-7_6

that has been mounting since before "this all began." Although I did not get my wish, I did take my first work call to encourage a colleague, Jim Knowles, to join the USC team. It was a small but important victory.

When I was moved to Cedars-Sinai on April 13th, the doctors concluded that I continued to have some difficulties with aphasia, right-side paresis, and other issues related to my left temporal and bilateral frontal lobe brain injuries. During the ambulance ride transferring me from USC, I once again implored the driver to just "drop me off" at home in Altadena. When I arrived at my room, I was confined to the bed and sedated to prevent further risk of injury. At this point, I'm told I was treating my injury like "old news." When the doctor held a mirror up to my head to show me a reflection of my dented skull where the bone was missing, I reluctantly conceded that one side was bigger than the other. On Friday, April 14th, I was presented with a wheelchair, somewhat to my displeasure. The rehab specialist assisting me in using it commented that I was persistent in getting what I wanted, to which I mischievously replied, "moi?" (who me?). After wheeling around for a few days, I was able to take my first steps without a walker but with the damn helmet and an aide's assistance (Fig. 6.1).

Amidst all of this progress, I was still impatiently and persistently requesting to go home. Poor Carlos took the brunt of it—on the chin. When discussing plans for the summer and future with my family, I declared, "Everyone should get what they want *except* Carlos." He wasn't succeeding in getting me home, so to hell with him!

In patients with TBI, frontal lobe injuries can result in uncharacteristically aggressive or disinhibited behavior. Often referred to as the leader, governor, or boss of the brain, any damage to the frontal lobe can affect a person's judgment and self-awareness. * My reaction to such a catastrophic injury was a pressing sense that I still had to manage and execute responsibilities, which was very much in character for me and a good sign for my recovery. However, to abate my anxiety, the medical professionals suggested assigning me tasks to assure me that work was, in fact, being completed. Having a 9 a.m. to 3 p.m. rehabilitation schedule of physical

Fig. 6.1 The hated helmet needed to get out of bed safely

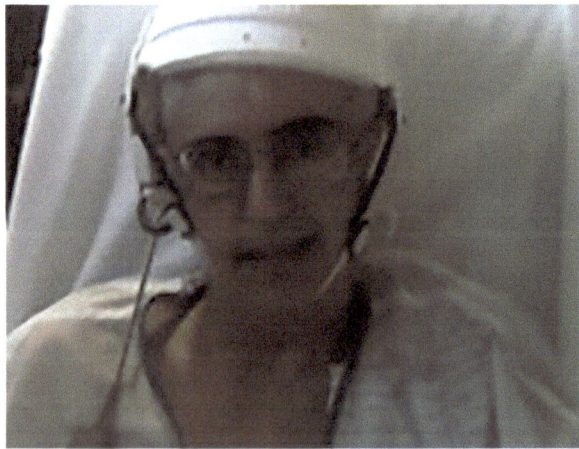

therapy, cognitive therapy, and speech therapy gave my days more structure and something productive "to do." I can't recall the extensiveness of the rehab while in the hospital; however, I pushed the limits of my rehab so much that on April 17th, my family, the Tortoras, described my wheelchairing as Tour de France training!

Despite my outward impatience, I do not remember a time where I felt pain or discomfort or was unable to accomplish a goal asked of me. If I was told to lift an object, I did. If I was told to place full weight on my legs, I did. It was frustrating, though, to be asked to practice doing very simple tasks as if no one trusted that I could keep myself in balance. I understood what people were saying to me and knew exactly what it was that I wanted to say in response, but the words leaving my mouth were not the ones that I was intending to speak. Not being understood, yet having my thoughts intact, was maddening. The funniest part of my language errors was that I constantly made reference to medical terms instead of everyday objects. I'm sure my language was even further behind than I was able to realize at the time, and it was only through the puzzled look on others' faces and Carlos's constant interpreting and corrections that my deficit was made known to me. For example, I was given a labyrinth exercise in rehab where I would trace the path to the end incorrectly, and then ask, "Right?" with a twinkle in my eye, still hoping I was correct. Like a child, I was searching for positive reinforcement in such tasks, as I couldn't judge yet what was correct.

Carlos might characterize things differently. Just days before I was released from the Rehab Unit, my therapist was putting me through the paces of daily living. She had me shower with her in the bathroom and go through the usual activities of self-grooming. One of the tasks was to brush my teeth. She asked me to and in response, I picked up a hairbrush, and the therapist noted on the record that I was unable to understand the command. Carlos had a different approach. He would say I understood brush, but he asked me to brush my teeth. This gave me encouragement that I was partially understanding the request but not the whole context, and it was a useful approach that acknowledged my personality. I sought to succeed, so the positive reinforcement with the immediate request to achieve the required task would work. I could then redirect myself and pick up the toothbrush. This pattern of positive reinforcement coupled with the expectation that I could and would do the task right helped push me to a much earlier recovery.

Looking back on this process, I would strongly suggest for anyone facing this kind of recovery from traumatic brain injury and for their families these two invaluable pieces of advice:

1. Try to be a patient patient.
2. Be a patient family member, friend, or medical caregiver with the patient.

As a doctor myself, I am well aware of the liabilities associated with giving overly optimistic prognoses, but I must say that the caregivers need better insight into their patients to know what their abilities were before the injury. For instance, when I was at Cedars-Sinai, I was terribly bored with the physical therapy rehabilitation. I had been in bed for 2 weeks, which was the most time in my life that I can recall ever not moving around. Even when I had chicken pox as a child, my mom would say that I refused to sit still. I bet moving around kept me distracted from itching and scratching myself! Working with the rehab therapists, I had to find a simple way to communicate my need for more physical stimulation. I would ask, "More times? How many? More tomorrow!" In the end, I continued to do more reps of that activity all day long just to stay active, given that my cognition wasn't yet up to speed. When the therapists returned the next day, I went beyond what they had scheduled. And, within a few days of this, they got the message, so to speak, and adjusted their physical rehab expectations based on what I had achieved from the day before. Even though TBIs often rob us of our means of expression, communicating your needs to the therapists, if even through others, is vital.

Bob and Lee Woodruff's book, *In an Instant: A Family's Journey in Love and Healing*, details how the journalist's family made all the difference in his own recovery from a TBI sustained by an IED explosion near Taji, Iraq. He received impeccable care but remained in coma for 40 days before waking up. https://www.brainandlife.org/articles/bob-woodruff-received-the-best-care-and-attention-after-a/

Ana astutely noted that my functionality and mood during this time improved dramatically whenever I was surrounded by close family and friends: I could recognize faces and speak more clearly.

My determined personality may have been frustrated with the rehab process, but it was also a blessing in disguise. If I hadn't been so adamant and eager to make progress, who knows if I would have been able to come as far as I did in such a short period of time. The resilience, or ability to bounce back, in a patient might have a direct correlation to their recovery's success. If there is such a thing as being well suited to the adversity of a TBI, perhaps I was because I had always pushed through mental and physical obstacles in the past. My physical stamina, which included running and doing 600 sit-ups a day, could have been the reason I sustained only minor lacerations on my liver and kidney and didn't bleed out or fully lose consciousness on the scene. Some believe that how you were before such a traumatic accident will determine how you will be after. Although there are exceptions, this is the hallmark of resiliency.

Having made so much progress in the hospital, on April 19th, it was determined by the neurosurgical doctors that I would be able to have my cranioplasty, the reconstructive surgery to replace my bone plate, in a matter of weeks. This is in spite of the practice guidelines that recommend 3–6 months (Fig. 6.2).

It was at this time that Carlos explained the situation to me. He had a lengthy conversation with me about my condition and the decisions that needed to be made in order to choose surgery or wait it out. *Oi!* He was pleased that I was able to provide very appropriate input to make the best decision. I told him, in my own way, that I would like to have the surgery to replace my bone and restore my skull as soon as possible. Medically speaking, the key to regaining my cognitive and linguistic functions would be restoring the existence of cerebrospinal fluid (CSF) pressure. Getting the normal flow of cerebrospinal fluid around my brain going would require that my skull would become a closed cavity again rather than the open one. One way to describe the situation is to imagine a drinking straw with a puncture that causes a

Fig. 6.2 Just 19 days after injury, look at the dent in my head!

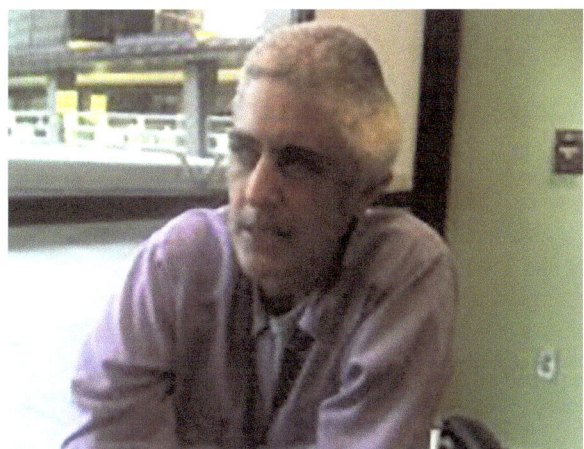

Fig. 6.3 Out to dinner, day 27, the day before the bone is put back

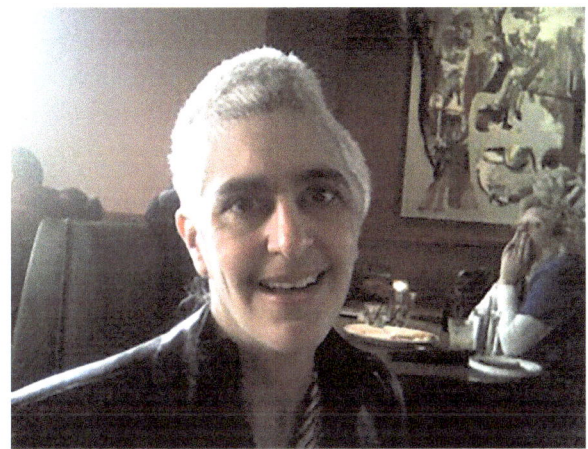

leak. Without a closed system, the straw becomes useless. The same applies for pressure in airplane cabins and space rockets (Fig. 6.3).

If my MRI indicated that the intracranial swelling continued to go down, I would have that surgery on April 28th, earlier than the doctors planned and the rehabilitation team of doctors recommended. As previously mentioned, it is unusually quick after performing a hemicraniectomy to reconstruct the skull within 1 month. According to practice guidelines and the rehabilitation team, they would recommend waiting as long as another 5 months.

Tongue-Tied

7

A pessimist sees the difficulty in every opportunity, while the optimist sees opportunity in every difficulty.

—Winston Churchill

Thus, the feeling I sometimes have – which all of us who work with aphasiacs have – that one cannot lie to an aphasiac. He cannot grasp your words, and cannot be deceived by them; but he grasps with infallible precision, namely, the expression that goes with the words....

—Oliver Sacks, author and neurologist

With the clock ticking down to my scheduled surgery in less than 10 days, there were two main goals for my recovery: first, to monitor the edema, or swelling, of my brain and, second, to continue an aggressive inpatient rehabilitation schedule. At this point, despite my constant pleadings to go home, I was stuck coping with the reality that I still had some proverbial mountains to climb at the hospital.

Therefore, I was immersed in daily sessions of speech and language therapy. I appeared to suffer from acute *anomic aphasia*, which is when it's challenging to name objects or find words. My family tells me that at times I would display more extreme deficits as I was becoming tired. Sometimes the fatigue would overcome me, and as I struggled to find the "right" words, I would express that exhaustion and reluctantly request a break so I could rest in my room. This was significant, since I always want closure and tend not to stop until I'm done. Additionally, self-monitoring was a very good sign in my healing because it showed that I was regaining some of the regulatory functions within my brain. Again, many TBI survivors suffer from disinhibition and lack self-control or awareness, and some never fully regain it. As I was relearning how to speak, my family had to learn how to communicate with me more effectively. They recognized that I required detailed descriptions of what was happening, cues on how to act, and they continually adjusted their expectations of me. They had to become more patient and judicious, as I often would become frustrated with myself for not communicating what I meant and with them for not understanding me.

Since my surgery was now imminent, Ana planned to come out to California to help both me and her brother Carlos, with my immediate postoperative recovery, from April 27th through May 1st. This is a great example of how the family support system becomes involved in the patient's recovery but also in helping other family members with their recovery. She vividly remembers the phone conversation we had when she told me of her trip to come see me.

I recognized Ana's voice and greeted her with, "Hi there!". I'm sure I could not remember her name, but I knew who she was in every other sense. Then, I asked about her two daughters and wondered what they were up to—school, plays, and birthdays coming up. I had some trouble fishing for their names and pertinent details but was able to get my questions across through trial and error. She remembers that I suggested her family should move out to Los Angeles! I reasoned that if her daughter Jillian was turning 7, she would be starting middle school soon and that's a good time to move. She let the miscalculation slide, since middle school would actually begin at age 11. I also called Chris, her husband, and her "son"! Her daughters then joined in, and although I was unable to remember their names, I spoke softly and appropriately to each of them. My 3-year-old niece Diana asked the question, "Why did you get squished by a car?" I explained in very lighthearted way that, "I don't know, maybe the car got *bored*!"

After the call, Ana tried to understand what I meant by "bored." It occurred to her that I was reaching for a word and that in many of our past conversations about the children's performances in school, words like "bored" were often used in conjunction with "distracted" or "inattentive." It clicked: what I was saying was that the car (or driver) was bored (distracted/inattentive).

Patients with the kinds of organizational deficits common in traumatic brain injury need to relearn a program of steps for every action, accommodating impairments they may have. In many cases like mine, you have to rebuild what were previously very automatic tasks. One example is the kind of neuromuscular memory required to serve a tennis ball or play an instrument. Once mastered, these motions become second nature. Your hands coordinate to toss up and then hit the tennis ball, and your fingers fall into place on piano keys. Traumatic brain injuries disrupt these ingrained processes, so the patient must reconnect the gaps by breaking down the action into minute steps. Brain injuries can affect many vital areas of the brain, so the tasks we need to retrain ourselves in will vary. In my case, the injury caused some right-side paresis, so I needed to focus on regaining strength on that side and on coordination. Although I was particularly gung ho and aggressive in my rehabilitation goals, it is important that TBI patients become flexible in their expectations and treat themselves with kindness.

It may be helpful to follow the well-known SMART system* of goal setting and achievement, which establishes that each goal (or task) must be:

Specific (answer the six "w" questions: who, what, where, when, which, and why)
Measurable (how much, how many, when will you know it's been accomplished?)
Attainable (plan your steps and establish a timeframe)
Realistic (being *willing* and *able* to achieve goal)
Timely (establish a firm deadline; not just "someday")

Rehabilitative specialists often recommend that TBI survivors take notes as they work toward their goals. To this day, I still rely on extensive notetaking to retain new facts or remember dates or appointments. As a med student, even before my head injury, I was always in the front row taking copious notes with my four-color Bic pen. But, it was only after my injury, that I realized how critical writing things down by hand has been in my learning, past and present. Now I take notes guilt-free and teach a class on how the neuromuscular act of writing aids memory.

Luckily, and perhaps also key to my recovery, I was able to continue interacting socially with my friends and family. When dining in the cafeteria with my family, I left the wheelchair behind. I was finally given "furlough" from the hospital for an evening so Carlos and I could have dinner out with our old friends, the Rappaports, Mark and Jacqueline. We have a long professional relationship with Mark, who had been in research training with us at the National Institute of Mental Health (NIMH) from 1986 to 1990. He was also a frequent collaborator on our genetics projects even though we have never worked at the same institution since our time at NIMH. It also happened that he was the first "babysitter" to our eldest child, Michael. He took care of Mike at 3 months of age so we could go out to dinner, baby-free, for our sixth wedding anniversary. Right after the accident, Mark, the then-Chair of Psychiatry at Cedars Sinai in Los Angeles, arranged for my transfer there from USC University Hospital. In addition, it was Jacqueline who gathered the seed pearls and amethysts from the three-strand necklace I was wearing during the accident and then repaired it for me. It's one of my favorite necklaces that I still wear today.

For dinner, we ate somewhere near the hospital, me with helmet on, and I recall asking for psychotherapy for my entrée, by accident, instead of spaghetti. This was a big deal: I could read the menu and enjoy the night out.

I was fortunate that I was allowed these sorts of daily field trips away from the hospital, albeit only with the helmet! The doctors would not allow me to go home overnight until the surgery to reconstruct my skull was scheduled. In fact, there was a bit of squabbling between the neurosurgeons and rehab doctors about whether it was too soon to perform the surgery at all. Carlos sided with the surgeons and felt confident they were making the right decision to move forward this quickly. The surgeons understood how important it was for me to have the repair completed as soon as possible. At the very least, I felt that it was psychologically beneficial to be allowed to do more and that I would have to be limited, for my safety, until the repair was complete. This did not sit well with the rehab therapists/physicians who advocated the following practice guidelines: waiting 3–6 months to replace the skull bone as a less risky treatment plan. While they acknowledged that Carlos was a doctor, they felt he was biasing his decision as my husband who wanted to please his wife. In addition, I was so desperate to go home! Without the intact skull, it would have been even harder for me to be at home for an extended number of hours unsupervised. What if I fell, with no bone to protect my brain, and no one was there to help me or call an ambulance?

It wasn't just that I was incessantly complaining about wanting to leave the hospital, but wearing the helmet was an impossible impediment. With the minimal protection it could provide, I wasn't able to do much of the physical activity I was used to. As a very active child, some would say I was a little too squirmy or hyperactive. ADHD, which wasn't often acknowledged when I grew up, could still come with high intelligence and good school performance. Therefore, to harness my "squirmy" disposition, vigorous exercise helped me focus. If I wasn't doing homework, then I was playing soccer or tennis. Then, running became my go-to physical activity once I was in medical school, and I stuck with it in the decades since. However, running was understandably a no-no with my hemicraniectomy and exposed brain. In addition, the helmet just wouldn't protect me enough if I fell. Bottom line, any daily physical activity made me feel more like myself. It grounded and focused me physically and mentally, and there were a limited number of physical activities I could do with the helmet compared to what I would be able to do with my skull intact. Carlos knew this, and so regardless of the opinion of the rehabilitation specialists, he pushed forward with the neurosurgeon's assessment to perform the cranioplasty (skull repair) because he believed it would aid my overall recovery.

Carlos saw his own physician for a checkup while I was still hospitalized and found that his blood pressure and EKG were the best it's been in years. His big joke was probably because he had no nagging wife at home. Nevertheless, he wanted me to get back to being myself; the sooner I got back to the things I liked, the better things would be.

However, ever since the accident, Carlos was battling bouts of insomnia as stress continued to mount. Some of it was based on the practical concern of moving and making our new home ready for my return. More troubling, he was also grappling with how unclear the new future was: how would I adapt to home life? Would I ever work again? This would be the first time Carlos would need to take on a caregiving role, which is an intimidating prospect for any spouse. I was still ornery with Carlos if he was not quick enough to "fix" my aphasic errors, so what would it be like for him to take care of me full time?

On April 21st, Carlos's parents arrived and were very happy to see the progress I made. Odette described me as "quite the handful." To them, I seemed very childlike and uncooperative with what the doctors *didn't* want me to do. They were anxious that I was moving about so quickly while my skull was open and brain was, essentially, exposed, especially Odette, Carlos's mother, who had been an obstetrical nurse and was pointedly used to dealing with new babies and postpartum mothers, many of whom, although not all, are very compliant with doctor's orders—especially with the first baby. The next day, on my son Michael's birthday, my family reported that my head became caved in, which was a sign that the swelling had gone down dramatically. I could walk and speak relatively normally, and my only obvious neurological problem was my continued aphasia.

A short glossary of my most common aphasic terms:

patients, students = "children"
shoes, clothes = "shirts"
foods = "berries" or "meds"
Carlos = "stupid"
emotions = "sexy"

Whenever Carlos tried to understand what I meant to say, I would either validate him or else say "stupid!" if it was wrong. It wasn't that I was calling him stupid, although it's possible he thought that in the moment! Rather, it was my way of saying that the word was stupid, and I was still searching for how to express myself.

On April 23rd, I was allowed to go home for a BBQ dinner. Carlos remembers that I coached *him* on how to drive home in the car. We also invited a research colleague and friend over to our house, and I decided that I wanted to make a fruit cobbler for the occasion. Carlos and Eric then took me grocery shopping, which was a challenge since my vocabulary was still riddled with aphasias. They would ask, "What kind of fruit do you need?" "Berries." Then, Carlos picked up berries, and I said "No, not those!" I *knew* exactly what I needed, but when I spoke, "berries" became many items on my list. They decided to march me up and down each aisle to allow me to select the ingredients on my own. It was a clever solution to my berry problem. Despite my language barrier, I was still very competent in the kitchen: I could cut, bake, manage the oven temperature, and execute my recipes.

I continued to use certain replacement words frequently: berries, meds, psychotherapy, cognitive behavioral therapy, and sexy. Ana tells me that during this time, I had a very positive attitude for trying out skills and that my reasoning was that I wanted to determine what I could and could *not* do. Unless I tested the skills out, I would have no idea what I needed to work on in rehab. I also became more anxious to know when it might be safe for me to go running.

With only 2 days until the scheduled surgery on April 28th, Carlos welcomed Ana to our new home in Altadena. I was also discharged that morning from Cedars-Sinai and then taken to USC for my final MRI in advance of my procedure there. When I arrived home, our house was practically bare; the furniture was supposed to arrive the next week. Ana observed that I was walking with no visible falter, limp, or hesitations. Without my helmet on, the dent in my head looked extreme. It appeared as though an almost 90-degree slice had been taken out of the left side of my skull. I was able to think critically and carry on conversations, which astounded Ana. It seemed implausible; it could take a long time before one of my symptoms surfaced. I wanted to convince the *other* medical professionals that I could go home, so I was overcompensating to present a good front.

Ana and I spent some quality time together away from the hospital, which was the first we had seen each other face to face since before the accident. We looked through a photo album of family pictures she brought, and I was able to remember everyone along with many of the events. Names, however, were tougher to recall. We went to the mall in Pasadena and shopped for hats. I was able to pay for my own purchase without help. However, as I became more tired and hungry, my aphasia and memory lapses (for distant events) became more pronounced. As fatigue set in, more confusion manifested. While we ate sushi, I received a phone call from Suzi, my sister. Afterward, though, Ana noticed I was confused about who it had been that I had talked to. While telling a story about Carlos's parents, I forgot that they were also Ana's parents. Ana gently explained that they were brother and sister and that meant they had the same parents.

After a late night, I slept in until 10 a.m. on April 27th and was able to pick out a yogurt and coffee for breakfast all by myself. Ana helped me with a load of laundry, and I was able to fold up the clothes neatly and with great attention to detail. Our only slip up was when we noticed that we forgot to read the labels and laundered "dry clean only" items. We spent the morning making a list for grocery shopping, which took longer than usual, about 2 hours.

It was a very "sexy" day at our home. This is because I continuously used the word "sexy" to describe when things were stupid, funny, silly, yummy, pleasant, embarrassing, or pretty. This was very amusing to my family members! "Berry" or the plural "berries" was also frequently used to describe food items, books, utensils, and other basic objects. Essentially, the go-to adjective was "sexy" and the fail-safe noun was "berry," so I ended up calling many things "sexy berries." Alternatively, I referred to condiments, jewelry, and small items as "meds" while deferring to the previously used "psychotherapy" for anything related to work, rehab, or school. I mislabeled my relatives by calling husbands "sons" and sisters "daughters."

Since the house and kitchen were brand new to me, we rearranged the refrigerator shelves and items by size or item type. This thorough exercise showed that my OCD tendencies remained intact! My main concern, which I expressed to Ana, was that we make room for "berries."

Later that day, I managed to prepare a steak and cheese tortilla lunch for everyone. I'm told they were sloppy but very tasty. I only broke one egg and got a small burn on my arm in the process, which wasn't that far below average, all things considered.

Then, we went grocery shopping, and my son Eric was very doting toward me. He took me by the arm and guided me up and down the aisles. Everything that went into the cart was a "berry," and sometimes I chose items for their attractive packaging than actual need. Ana's favorite moment of the trip was passing a display of bagged dried fruits, and I pointed and squealed, "Berries!" with surprise. Sure enough, this time it was bag of dehydrated berries. They did a double take (after all, everything up to this point was a berry) and burst out laughing.

Afterward, we sat on the outdoor furniture, waiting for Carlos to pick us up. I was very anxious and worried that something might have happened to him. When we returned home, I took a nap.

Putting the house in order continued to be a focus, and later we all went furniture shopping for a television stand. We went to a store that had multiple television screens on at once. I was overwhelmed by visual images, noise, and the crowd. As we continued on to another store, I decided that I had too much, so I just turned on my heels while Carlos was speaking to a clerk and started to walk out. Eric and Ana rushed after me. I was sitting on a bench outside. I asked Eric to get the keys so we could sit instead inside the car. It became clear to everyone that I was very fatigued. Ana saw my hands trembling and wondered if I might also be hungry.

On the way home, Carlos was having fun retelling an old story about getting his wisdom teeth pulled while he was in college, and I asked him where he went to school. He answered, "Brown." Then, I asked, "Where did I go to college?" Thankfully, once reminded, I was better able to recover these memories, and of attending Brown too!

Suzi called me that evening to wish me good luck, and although I was improving, she noticed that I was still mixing up words and my affect was a bit off. I thanked her for calling but didn't seem to truly take in why she was calling or wishing me "good luck" regarding the surgery. I was just so anxious (and perturbed) to get my skull plate back in place so I could run again.

The neurosurgeons evaluated my last MRI, performed on April 26th when I left Cedars-Sinai Hospital, which showed that the areas of swelling on the brain were decreasing satisfactorily. Despite any previous misgivings, I was "green-lighted" for my cranioplasty to take place early in the morning of April 28th (Figs. 7.1 and 7.2).

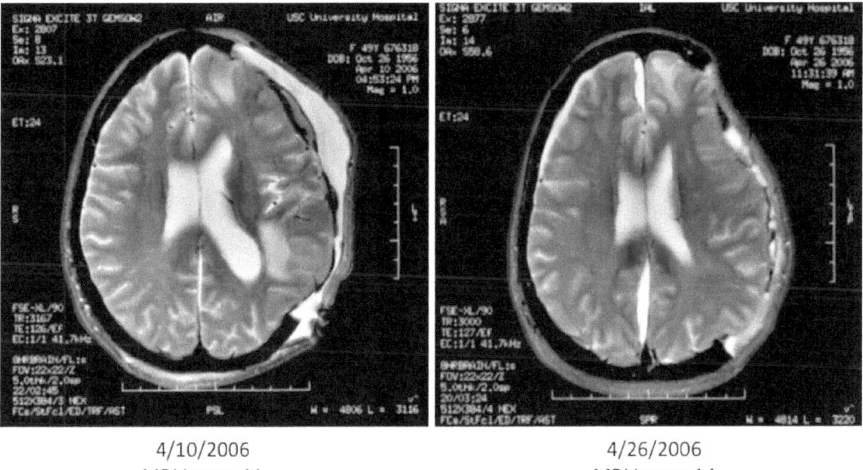

| 4/10/2006 | 4/26/2006 |
| MRI Image 11 | MRI Image 14 |

Fig. 7.1 The MRI before and after to how swelling decreased in just 16 days in the lateral ventricles and brain tissue, but the bone was not back yet!

Fig. 7.2 Further MRI
evidences the blood clot
(hematoma) was almost
gone, and the swelling of
3rd ventricle was less

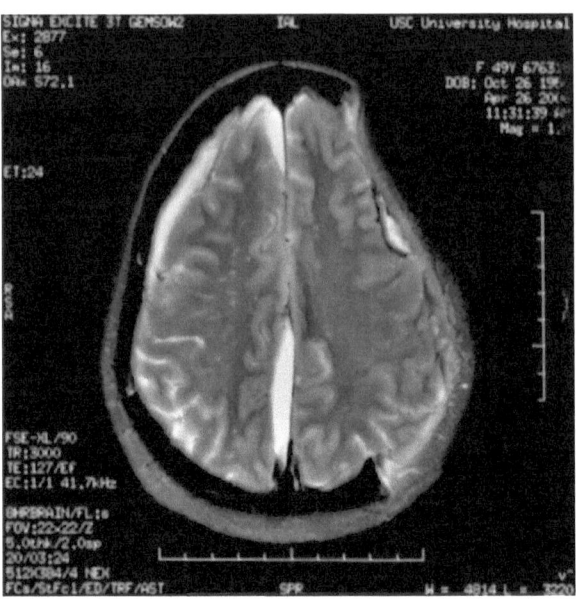

Stitches and Glue

8

Who looks outside, dreams; who looks inside, awakes.

—*Carl Jung, psychiatrist*

Paradoxically, we achieve true wholeness only by embracing our fragility and sometimes, our brokenness.

—*Jalaja Bonheim, author*

As I went off to surgery at USC, Carlos went off to work. The cranioplasty took more than 3 hours, which was longer than the neurosurgeons had initially expected. This made Carlos very nervous, but what else could he do but go to work? His office was right next to the hospital, and he tried to keep busy until they called him to say that I was out of the OR.

During the procedure, it became clear that the swelling of my brain was more significant than the last MRI had shown. They gave me a steroid and an injection of mannitol, a diuretic, to further reduce the brain fluid immediately before placing the bone in position and closing my skull. I was then moved to the ICU for recovery.

When my family was allowed to visit, they saw my skull intact for the first time in 4 weeks (Fig. 8.1). Ana observed that I looked "all fixed up" with a nice smooth, round shape. She was also surprised to hear that my voice, which she described as having had an "airy, childlike" quality before the surgery, is now completely back to my normal pitch and tone. My son Eric theorized that perhaps without the bone above my ear, I had found the sound of my voice too loud or resonant and therefore had adjusted it to a comfortable pitch. I remember immediately requesting the telephone so that I could call my father and let him know I was okay. When I called and he picked up in New York, I said, "Hi, Dad, it's Michele." He replied, "No kidding!" and "I know, you sound like yourself again!" Finally, my voice matched my thoughts. When my voice changed from soprano to alto in puberty, it had taken on some of the deeper resonant quality of my southern Italian dad, and I guess he was

M. T. Pato, *Nerve*, https://doi.org/10.1007/978-3-031-33433-7_8

Fig. 8.1 I wake up in recovery, bone is back in place (cranioplasty), and I want to go home

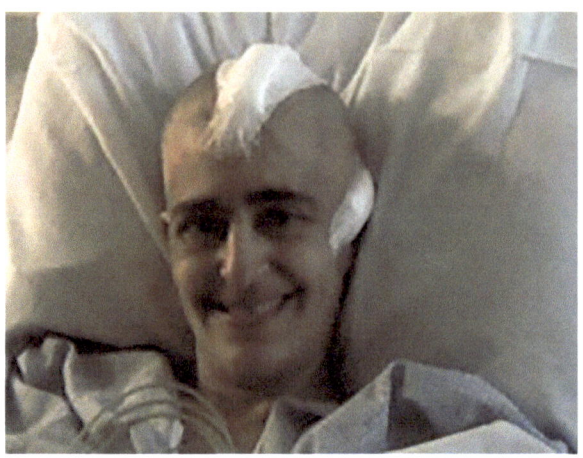

glad to have the "ole Michele" back. We had shared this vocal connection since I was an adolescent, a similarity, and it was now restored, which I'm sure was deeply comforting to him as it was to me. It was probably my second full sentence since my TBI on April first, the first one being when I asked the nurses in recovery, "Can I please have a phone?"

I was very uncomfortable in the ICU while attached to tubes and a catheter in my bladder. I fussed about my IV, worried that it might get a kink in it. The attending nurses assured me many times that it was okay, but I was unconvinced. My main interests were getting something to drink and something to eat and, of course, getting out of the hospital as soon as possible. Suzi noted, "This was an ongoing agitation of yours that was practically in every sentence you spoke regarding when you could resume your normal activities. It was so *you* to be onto the next step, regardless of what was truly going on medically. You were not focusing on the seriousness of your medical condition, for, of course you would heal, and instead you were focusing on getting back to your routines".

My family left me to rest for the evening. Now the next step was getting paroled, sent home from the hospital!

The next day, on April 29th, I was discharged from USC at 1 p.m. I was very concerned about my getting prescriptions in order, and so we went straight from the hospital to the pharmacy. The doctors put me on a low dose of Keppra, an epilepsy medication, to prevent future seizures. I was also very preoccupied with getting back on my birth control medication. Many around me were not surprised that I wanted to demonstrate "good patient" behavior and take my medicines, but everyone smirked a bit, and I do now looking back on it, about why I wanted the birth control pill started immediately. Honestly, I think it was a good sign about my recovery. First, as a pragmatist I didn't want to get pregnant, I had friends who were as old as 45 or 50 when had their first child and so biologically I knew it wasn't impossible, and honestly I didn't want my recovery to be even more complicated. However, by now, it had been 1 month since I had had sex with my husband. That was a long time for us, and I didn't want any further delay. However, no matter how organized my thoughts were about the issue at the time, as soon as I got home, I was tired and had to take a nap straight away.

I learned quickly that I had to modify or censor myself to avoid trouble in conversation. Instead of speaking a lot, I decided to just listen to ongoing conversation from time to time. I would often excuse myself quickly from telephone calls with family and friends in order not to make a mistake or misspeak. When Carlos interviewed a woman to do housekeeping, I had to walk away from the interview. However, afterward, I told Carlos exactly what I thought. I suggested we needed someone more competent and that we needed to find a service so that we could have background and reference checks done and hire someone responsibly. I'm not sure exactly how I was able to express myself, but he told me his interpretation and I said "yes," very relieved he understood.

That first evening home, I decided that I wanted to go out to eat for dinner. Eric drove the car for practice. Ana, seeing that I was unnerved by every driver on the road, wondered if I may have any PTSD from the accident, but one of the fortunate aspects of a severe TBI is that you lose the memory of the incident entirely. I don't recall the cars colliding or being hit at all, so I believe it was more likely me being a nervous backseat driver with a relatively "new" driver like Eric. To be honest, they (mom, dad, Bryce, Paul, and Suzi) were all anxious about driving with Eric, who was overly cautious even after he received his license a year or two later. He did not regulate his speed well, often slowing down rather abruptly; he seemed to have difficulty with distance between cars; and most significantly, he made abrupt lane changes, which felt like right angles rather than lane shifts sometimes. I also wonder how nervous he must have been to be driving me on that first night after surgery. It is interesting that Carlos supported him doing this too; it might have been everyone's desire to get everything back to normal as soon as possible. For us, we wanted to let Eric know we trusted him. For Eric, he revealed to me that part of his difficulty with driving and the long road to getting his license at the end of college was due to having a strong, anxious fear of the lethal power of handling a motor vehicle after my injury. This further reinforces the fact that TBIs affect family members and loved ones in many different ways.

When we arrived at the nearby bistro, I was beginning to feel signs of fatigue and just nibbled on my food. As we sat in the outdoor courtyard, people we knew stopped by to say hello. At this point, I was speaking with very few aphasic errors. Nevertheless, I was having trouble following the conversation, and when I felt too tired to continue socializing, I asked the waiter for the check. Meanwhile, back at the house, my mother had arrived by taxi from the airport. Since Ana could only stay with us for about a week, she would be leaving soon, so my mom came out to help. Family and friends are crucial because they know what you were like before the accident. Not only do they help you remember the past, but you tend to trust them more than the rehab therapists whom you have never met before.

We took many walks as a family. For lunch the next day, Carlos drove me, Eric, Ana, and my mother to Malibu for a breakfast buffet at a restaurant called Gidget's, and then we went for a walk on the boardwalk there. Back at home I rested, but opted not to nap. Later, Ana and I walked through my running route in the

Fig. 8.2 Had to stay
overnight but yeah home
the next day in street
clothes!

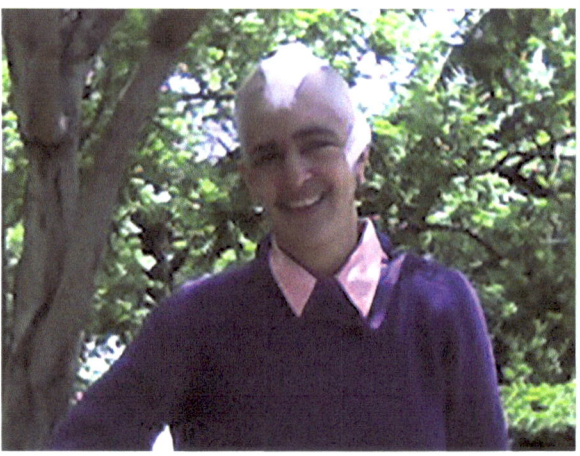

neighborhood. Back in March, before my TBI, I had gone on a few runs here, and I was able to remember the specific directions. Luckily, even after the TBI, my sense of navigation remained intact (Fig.8.2).

However, the more tired I became, the more Ana noticed my symptoms surface. I would begin to lose patience with the amount of time it took to do things, and I would become quiet when I caught myself using the wrong word. With all of these adjustments to process, I continued to think about what I might need to be doing next to speed up my recovery along. And, as Suzi says, "Michele has always been about speed and efficiency." It's good to know some things hadn't changed!

One of the other negative symptoms I experienced and that my family endured was a tendency to obsess about one issue. As Eric was not returning to school but finishing out his senior year of high school from California, I became fixated on whether or not he was doing his homework. This extra attention also put stress on him.

Because there was an extreme difference in the way I functioned when my energy was high versus when it was running low, that change took a toll on Carlos. Although I know I tried hard to act my best 100% of the time, that was an impossible expectation. As with any recovery process, there would *have* to be low points in order to discover how to navigate through what I needed in terms of rest and pacing.

When Ana left to go home on May first, she recorded her thoughts about her time with me and tried to process what she witnessed. It strikes me how profound and impactful one person's injury can be on many people. No one is untouched by a loved one's TBI. Ana wrote:

> I find that the enormity of this situation floods me with emotions. Joy, gratitude, incredulousness, wonder, amazement, concern for the future, a desire to continue to help, slight mourning for a past left behind, but mostly an energized hope that expectations will continue to be exceeded.
>
> I hope I have been some help. I am glad to have the chance to clear my mind before arriving back home. It is impossible to go through this experience without feeling somehow changed.

Even as I felt the sobering weight of the reality that my brother's and nephew's lives were now forced into a different shape than they had been in the years leading to Michele's accident, I couldn't help but feel a tugging hope for the future. I had been made conscious of the elegance in mental processing while watching Michele work to regain hers. Observing Michele apply direct attention to the task of slicing a vegetable, for example, in incremental steps from the planning to the execution, made me aware of how infrequently we remain mindful about the tasks we set out to accomplish. The Zen-like quality of moving with Michele through life, one contemplative moment at a time, was an inadvertent gift for me. I have clung to this awareness from that day on.

Hands

9

Our moving truck from Bethesda broke down in transit, so we were living in a house without furniture. As a result, there was a state of chaos apart from my recovery in those early days of May. People were constantly coming and going, Carlos was in full swing at work, and we had little more than a few boxes to remind us of home. During that time, I was able to accompany Carlos to work functions such as his Grand Rounds lecture at USC and recruitment dinners, where I wore stylish hats to disguise my injury. However, things were far from normal.

My recovery plan forbade me from doing all sorts of perfunctory tasks that a move requires: bending down, lifting boxes, and any activity that could put me at risk for a fall, which could then induce bleeding. When you are a newly released TBI patient, your chances of reinjuring your head are significant and carry dire consequences. Yet my brain, perhaps a bit bullish and disinhibited, ironically wanted to do it all. Carlos remembers that when no one (Eric, my mother, or rehab therapists) was looking, I would go move boxes and try to unpack. He thought having movers come and unpack would be a good idea, but it left a gigantic mess that I felt unable to leave alone. In many cases, my family tells me, I had become uncooperative and frustrated (and frustrating). When given the task of deciding which things from our old home to throw away, I often threw the baby out with the bath water, so to speak. Unsatisfied with my occupational rehabilitation, which I believed totally useless, I even tried to terminate this aspect of the rehab. The Pato home was tense, patience went out the window, and my mother even began to feel that her opinions were unwelcome. As an anxious person, this was not so unusual, even less so for an Italian-American Long Islander. She has strong opinions and often interjects her ideas whenever she feels they are needed. During this visit, she noticed our difficulties and wanted to help but felt helpless given the tension in the environment, which made her even more worried. I also wonder if she was triggered psychologically. After all, she was at the scene of the accident and witnessed everything firsthand. As a child, she endured her younger sister's polio affliction and rehabilitation, which was no doubt traumatic for her. In addition, here I was, a 50-year-old woman trying to show my mother that her adult daughter could "do it" and make my own decisions.

I realize now that we tried to muddle through what was a near impossible task: get me on track with proper outpatient and in-home therapies while in the throes of moving. We had no choice, truly, due to the unpredictability of events, but it made an already stressful time worse. Carlos complained that I was doing too well but not well enough. He still feared that I might crash and burn at any moment. My disinhibition caused by the damage to my frontal lobe made for possibly tense social exchanges, and at one recruitment dinner I attended with Carlos, I made a faux pas with a colleague by talking about changes to the residency training I planned to make though I hadn't officially been assigned that task yet. What I saw as eagerness to get involved and back to work was interpreted by some who barely knew me as "taking over." Not the best way to start a new job!

Luckily, and I cannot emphasize this enough, I had lots of people around me to lend a hand and help our family out. They knew me. Most had known me for many years before my injury, so even when the right words didn't come out, or I was rough or unfiltered, they could interpret it in a way that they understood what I meant.

Helena, our longtime family friend and research colleague, made the move from her home in Massachusetts to work with us in California. She had already agreed to follow us to USC. However, after the accident happened, she was even more resolved that she was needed.

I first met Helena back in 1993 when I took the job of Medical Director at the Corrigan Mental Health Center in Fall River, Massachusetts. At that time, she was the Clinical Chief of the bilingual Portuguese-English mental health workers. Then, in 1997, when our research grant came through, we went to visit the Azores and coincidentally ran into Helena, a native Azorean who was visiting her family. We asked her then if she would like to join the study. She accepted, and we have been working with her ever since. Initially, the job required her to travel between the United States and the Azores, overseeing diagnostic interviews and collecting blood samples of the study's participants. She was the perfect fit to bridge the language and culture gap and to run our clinical laboratory studies there for several years before returning to the United States to do ongoing work on them. It was easy for Carlos to connect to their shared Portuguese heritage, and we considered her part of the family. Affectionately referred to as "Tia Helena," she watched our boys grow up and had keys to our various homes over the decades we have worked together.

Shortly after Helena arrived in Altadena, California, the truck transporting our furniture and remaining boxes finally appeared from Maryland. As we did with all of our major moves (14 and counting!), we had the movers pack everything up from the old house and place the furniture and boxes in "their" rooms in the new house. We'd also rented a large dumpster to throw out things that didn't fit into the new house or that we didn't need anymore. This method of moving, which had worked so well for us in the past, became much more complicated with my injury. Helena stepped in to arrange with the movers in Bethesda, Maryland, and made what would have been an impossible move possible. She had not seen our new house, so boxes which would have been labeled and placed just so in "master bedroom," "guest room," "office," and so on could not be labeled the way I would have done it. She did her best, but my compulsively organized personality was thrown into hyperdrive.

Although I was limited in what I was allowed to do, getting the kitchen up and running to my standards were a top priority. After spending years cooking side-by-side with me making Portuguese and Italian dishes in several of my kitchens, Helena felt assured that she could assist me in setting this one up. However, before Helena could go to work unloading the kitchenware boxes, I had pushed my way through and started the process myself, strictly against doctor's orders. If I lowered my head, the balance of pressure and circulation to my brain could change, creating a life-threatening situation. And, despite pleadings from others, I frequently brushed off admonitions by asserting, "I'm fine, I'm fine." Although not my intention, my responses to friends and family could come off as very angry and dismissive. The natural reaction would be for the person to get angry in return; however, they might remind themselves that I was still recovering. Not an easy task in the heat of the moment! My denial could have been seen by some as a very healthy defense mechanism that helped to advance my recovery by engaging in low-risk activities. To others, however, what they saw was my injured frontal lobes impairing my judgment.

On a positive note, before I made more language missteps, I began to say, "I can't think of the word for" this or that. There was still a struggle to remember where to locate my things or how to operate the appliances in the new house. Aside from trying to find the correct words for items, I was also faced with determining where they might be! I would reach for a cup or bowl that used to be in a cupboard above the stove, but instead my mother or Helena stacked them on a shelf near the refrigerator. Making new memories was a challenge, and it took me a long time to learn where everything was now located. It was difficult to feel settled and at home. It wasn't truly my home yet, since I had never fully lived in it before my injury.

Oftentimes my son Eric, my mother, and Helena felt like they were given an impossible task: to save me from myself. In my mind, it was only natural to push back on those trying to set limits because all I wanted to do was reestablish my autonomy. As I continued to progress, I wanted even less of others' help.

Carlos too did not want me to be overly coddled and knew that excessive attempts to limit me for safety's sake could be received by me as reinforcing disability. He learned that it was a precarious balance to protect me but somehow remain hands-off enough so that I could regain full function and independence. In retrospect, I can see how he would insert himself as a buffer between myself and others to prevent unnecessary arguments. For example, I found my baptismal dress that we had kept for 50 years, and I was about to throw it into the dumpster. Helena stopped me, and I got angry saying, "When will I ever wear this again, it doesn't fit?"

The time it takes for any patient suffering from traumatic brain injury to recover proper judgment skills varies depending on the severity and location of the brain injury. The other factor is the patient's access to and quality of care. At the outset of my rehabilitation, I was assigned a team of specialists to assist me: a physical therapist, an occupational therapist, and a speech/language therapist. For weeks, I dutifully worked with these therapists at Rehab Without Walls, but as the time went on, I became increasingly worried about the professional obligations I was neglecting at work. To assuage my concerns, Carlos began to communicate with my colleagues about my work, and on May 8th, just 10 days after my skull repair, I emailed for the first time. I was even able to type at full speed. When asked what my next professional goal might be, I said, "To be Carlos's boss!" Funny, but true!

At this point, my day-to-day occupational goals were being met, and I kept asserting that I could do more than asked of me. According to the rehab schedule, I was assigned physical rehab for a total of 2 months, which was disappointing, since I believed I could get it done in one. On May 9th, Carlos sat in on my "assessment conference" to determine where I was in the process and to determine what I would still need going forward. The assessment concluded that my occupational/cognitive therapies were going well, and I needed another month of physical rehab where the therapist would run and swim with me. My weakness, of course, was my speech, and so that therapy would continue beyond all others.

Framed another way, once released from the hospital in the 7.5 weeks between May 1st and June 21, 2006, I had at least 41 appointments/sessions: 6 MD appointments, 11 Physical therapy sessions, 11 Speech and Language sessions and 13 Occupational therapy sessions.

As I was trying to reclaim my language skills and memory, Ana recalled that I would repeat the same stories over and over again perhaps because I didn't remember I had told it to that person or to anyone at all. Additionally, if I couldn't remember a person's name from the past, I might decide it was because they were "no good" or some brand of "not worth knowing." This may have been a mechanism that I developed to explain my memory issues, and I was oblivious to the harshness of what I was saying.

It became an emotional situation for Helena, and she confided in others that she felt ill-equipped to deal with some of the things that I was zinging at her. In one instance, I was throwing things out and accidentally threw away some of Helena's clothes. Looking back, I probably did not recognize the items and therefore made the connection that because they were unfamiliar, they weren't needed. In another flurry of unpacking, I also examined my wedding dress, which had also been my mother's wedding dress, thought there was no need to use it again (we had two boys, after all), and attempted to toss it in the dumpster. There was some rationale for my thinking, I believe, but the impulsive decisions I was making were jarring. This hit Helena particularly hard, and she perhaps took this as a personal slight. With tensions already high, she feared that we might not be able to reestablish our prior connection following the injury and even confided in Carlos at one moment that she thought she may not be able to continue with us professionally as our research coordinator. It became apparent that we needed some space between us to neutralize any possible resentment for my condition and behavior. Helena had always known me as a fair and forthright person, and now what she saw was a different version of me. Although this could well be temporary, that was not always easy to see in the moment. It's likely that I was too demanding without realizing how impaired I was at the time. Rather than wanting to rely on those around me, it was of utmost importance that I asserted my place. I pushed help away rather than appreciate the support being offered.

She also believed that I was pushing myself too hard and noticed that my face began to droop if I didn't rest. She wondered, what if I didn't meet my own arbitrary goals, would it be emotionally devastating to me? It must have been overwhelming for her, and so she decided to start the process of looking for a place nearby to live to give each other some more privacy and space.

With Helena moving out, on May 16th, Cindy Wojtecki, a former colleague and friend from Syracuse, New York, joined us in California. She was a VA nurse and frequent research collaborator of mine. We had been working on a journal article called "Teaching Interested Clinicians How to Develop Research Projects," which was up for publication in *Academic Psychiatry*. When Cindy heard about the accident, she retreated to her office as the Director of Education at Syracuse Veterans Administration, the news of my traumatic brain injury reducing her to tears. She had always known me to be full of energy and determination, appreciated my mentoring and guidance throughout the years, and it was heartbreaking to learn what had happened to me.

Cindy had accepted admission to the Nursing Ph.D. program at the University of California at San Francisco and was planning to make a temporary move from Upstate New York. With several of our projects and articles delayed due to my untimely injury, Carlos called Cindy and suggested that I hire her as she transitioned to California so that we could complete our projects together. Since Cindy knew me and my work so well, she was uniquely able to ease me back into it before I had to begin focusing on my responsibilities at USC. She agreed to come and stay with us for a month.

A couple of days later, on May 18th, my stitches were removed, and I was given instructions on how to clean the wound (Betadine and then Lubriderm) to allow it to properly heal. My physical therapy continued, though it was restricted to swimming and elliptical exercise. Always pushing forward, I made a deal with my son Mike that once I could run 3 miles again, then he would have to quit smoking. (It worked!)

Even though Carlos thought my outward recovery was going so well at this 6-week mark since my injury that you wouldn't know what had happened to me, the inner challenges persisted. A colleague from New York, who was a neuroscientist, came to visit and was very impressed with my condition. Despite everyone's appraisal that I was recovering beautifully, I was suffering from the dissatisfaction of not being able to work and with the disappointment of not being sure where my career would go next.

Having Cindy, a skilled nurse and natural caregiver, was comforting, but it was a role reversal we hadn't experienced before. Instead of mentoring her and driving the cowriting process, my aphasic errors made me take a backseat. All I could do was reject or approve drafts when shown to me and hope the next version would improve. Luckily, we ultimately pushed through and published the article on August 4, 2006, with the help of another colleague, Michael Wade, from the VA Center in Syracuse.

As the days passed, we caught up with life and its never-ending to-dos. I began the process to get my driver's license renewed, our house in Bethesda was sold and the closing papers needed to be signed, and Eric's high school graduation was coming up in June. We also had a grant in DC that needed to be renegotiated, so we decided to fly out on May 24th and handle the grant and the closing. It was a successful trip, though Carlos, with more responsibilities at work than ever before, was becoming exhausted.

We got to celebrate my progress over an extended Memorial Day weekend. My sister, Suzi, Paul, her son Bryce, and my parents came to California. It was special because with all of our moves around the country, we rarely got all together beyond the major holidays of Thanksgiving, Christmas, and Easter before the accident. Suzi visited me three times in 2 months (the week of the accident on April 1, Easter, and now Memorial Day). Of all those visits, this one was the most joyful and playful (Fig. 9.1).

Everyone was in a good mood for it was obvious that I was truly on the road to recovery. They even lovingly embraced my "know-it-all" need to be directing all activities, which was my hallmark before the accident. For them, it was so exciting

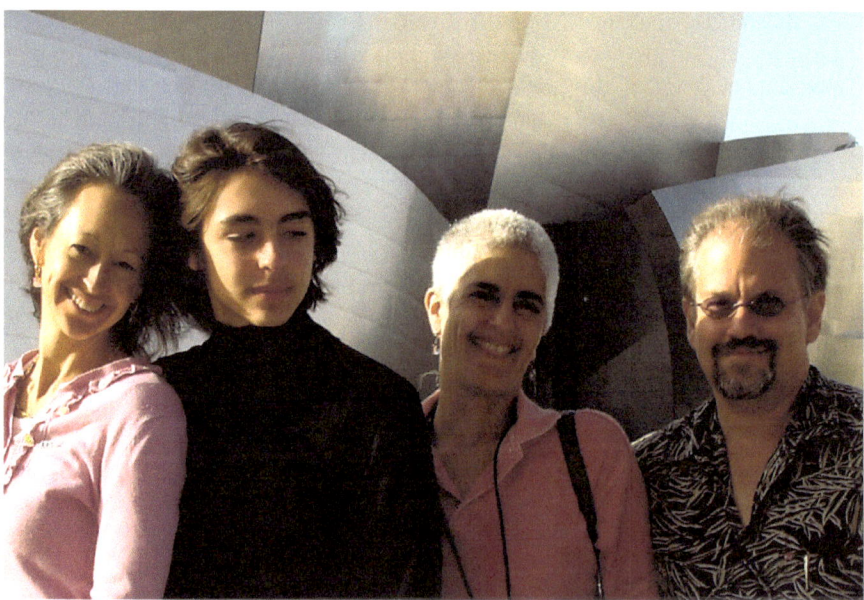

Fig. 9.1 A memorial day celebration with my sister and her son just 1 month after my bone is back and hair is growing

to see me regaining my sense of self in leaps and bounds. Although Suzi thought my progress was remarkable, she noticed that I was a bit childlike, my affect was off, I had an exaggerated smile, and I was unable to read social cues accurately. And, she noted that my mood could change very quickly, and I seemed mercurial. My family was very understanding about all of this for they were aware that I was still in the early stages of recovery. Although I don't remember this all that well, they observed that I was not sensitive to other people's emotions (what is called "reflective capacity" in infant mental health). I could be sweet and thoughtful in one moment but unable to empathize with others in the next.

When they arrived the afternoon of May 27th, I was receiving a PT treatment. Since Suzi is trained in dance and movement therapy, I was eager for her to observe my progress with the therapist. My stamina, accuracy, and strength were evident to her, and I was very pleased to show how well I could execute the given tasks. The next morning, I asked Suzi to escort me on my "run," which for the moment was a walk through the neighborhood. The house, a contemporary positioned high up on Glen Allen Lane in Altadena, was just steps away from the Angeles National Forest, filled with arid mountain trails and beautiful vistas. We hiked up this terrain together. Suzi was a bit concerned about the heat and the steepness of the path, but I looked at her like she was crazy and exclaimed, "What are you worried about?" As if it was Suzi who had an injury!

That evening, from our outdoor patio, pool, and upstairs windows, everyone marveled at the twinkling city lights of Los Angeles. Suzi remembers our home as a true oasis. The walls were gray, lavender, and sand stucco. There was a spacious open layout, two-story high ceilings and glass windows, doors, and stone floors, which created a seamless passage between the inside living space and outdoor patio garden. The airy patio also had two-story high beams and a ceiling that covered the outdoor kitchen and built-in BBQ. Beyond the slate patio was the large aqua blue swimming pool with a jacuzzi and stone path winding down the mountainside garden. As Suzi watched me over this whole weekend, she reflected on the spa-like atmosphere that must be contributing greatly to my healing. She could understand why I fought so hard to get out of the hospital to go home! Even though this was a new home, the beauty of the space, the sunlight, and the California weather as well as being surrounded by my loving family and friends were comforting and conducive to my recovery.

The second night, we barbecued, and I was totally involved. I confessed in passing that I had lost my sense of smell, but this does not stop me from cooking for 1 minute! My family ran over to the stove and oven from time to time to remind me that something smelled like it was burning! This just added to the festive atmosphere. Carlos manned the BBQ so that at least the main items of the meal were watched vigilantly. Carlos, a music lover, blared rock and roll on the outdoor sound speaker system. For the first time, we combined our passions—Suzi's being dance, and Carlos' being music, and we all danced as mom and dad watched. Paul, Suzi, and Bryce threw in some swing dance moves, and Carlos actually tried some of those moves out, too! It is the warmest, closest engagement Suzi has ever had with Carlos, and they both acknowledged how good it felt to be family. In spite of the present challenges we were all facing, it allowed us to become closer and even more bonded than ever before. It's important to feel joy and gratitude whenever you can.

Before the accident, Carlos and I had agreed to do a televised interview about our research program at USC that was scheduled for June. Although Carlos was now prepared to do it on his own, knowing me, he asked the interviewers to include me to the greatest degree possible. They all agreed that they could always edit the footage if necessary, although they never told me this before the interview. When the crew arrived at our labs at USC, I sat next to Carlos, and it became evident that I would not be sitting quietly and listening to him speak but as usual wanted to actively participate. As soon as the cameras rolled, like reciting a poem I knew by heart, I spoke fluently and responded to their questions with no aphasic errors. Carlos watched with amusement, as he saw me performing "onstage" for the first time since the accident. Carlos would chime in too, but he allowed me to shine. As the first question was asked, "Can you tell us about your research?" I jumped in, to say something like this (June 2006):

> We've actually been doing research in genetics in mental illness, specifically schizophrenia and bipolar disorder for our entire career. We've been practicing for approximately 20 to 25 years and we initially began with participants in Portugal.
>
> Carlos is bilingual; he lived in Portugal until he was 7, so we had some unique opportunities there. There are three major centers in Portugal, Lisbon, Coimbra, and Porto, and one colleague in particular was very interested in doing genetics work with us, so we offered to teach them more about genetics.
>
> After working a year or two on the mainland, they said to us, 'We should truly do this work in the Azores and maybe Madeira.' We immediately agreed. This gave us an opportunity to work with a homogenous sample because the Portuguese settled the Azores in the 1400s and there was no one there.

Although I battled through a few "uhs" and "ums" and was absolutely spent afterward, I had not made a mistake!

Carlos describes this video session as one where he let Michele take the lead fully expecting to have to do it himself after "letting her" try. He was amazed at her performance. Perhaps because this was a well-rehearsed presentation, she did not commit aphasic errors. Michele was proving herself professionally capable. She was clearly exhausted after less than 30 min of interview but had done it perfectly. Carlos told the film crew there was no need to do it over.

This was somewhat interesting since early on I called spaghetti "psychotherapy," but obviously, by this point, I was better able to retrieve memories and words associated with our life's work and speak about them without difficulty or error. Rather than the spontaneous, novel conversations I often struggled with after the injury, I had been a seasoned speaker in lectures and classrooms about our research and field of expertise. I had done this a thousand times before. In this arena, I could be responsive and fluid and recall statistics with accuracy. This development was the most important milestone thus far. In fact, Carlos felt I should return to work as soon as possible because it appeared to be an environment that I seemed almost better prepared to master than being at home.

Heart

It is not how much you do, but how much love you put in the doing.

—Mother Teresa, missionary

Family is not an important thing. It's everything.

—Michael J. Fox, actor and Parkinson's disease advocate

One of Carlos's most responsible steps in the early days after the accident was to seek out medical attention for himself. The stress of caregiving, sleeplessness, and worry about impending surgeries and unclear futures all contributed to extreme fatigue. Having medical knowledge does not necessarily make it easier. You may think of more things to worry about! Wear and tear on a person will result in health problems that could interfere with the ability to best provide for a loved one.

Below is part of a report written by professor, psychiatrist, and longtime friend Dr. S., who treated Carlos by phone for anxiety and post-traumatic stress disorder (PTSD) shortly after the accident. It reveals the immediate effects of the accident from Carlos's perspective and the subsequent stress he endured attempting to balance care between me and himself.

Massachusetts General Hospital/Harvard Medical School [letterhead]
When Carlos presented to me, he reported that he had flashbacks, nightmares, and intrusive, reexperiencing of the accident. Moreover, he experienced himself as hypervigilant, "on the edge," and had marked arousal when he encountered situations reminiscent of the accident. He had difficulty driving, with extreme difficulty "often taking approximately 10 minutes to drive through an intersection." Carlos reported experiencing emotional numbness, irritability, and hypervigilance. His startle reflex (particularly when anything entered his peripheral vision) was

M. T. Pato, *Nerve*, https://doi.org/10.1007/978-3-031-33433-7_10

extremely heightened, and he had difficulty concentrating. It was consistently reported by his colleagues that he was distracted at work.

Carlos also exhibited repeated emotional distress, heart palpitations, and shortness of breath and experienced his chest as tight when he reexperienced (internal or external) reminders of the accident. These symptoms are common post-traumatic stress symptoms, but in Carlos's case, they did not evolve into panic attacks.

Carlos also suffered from vegetative signs of depression, which included sleep disturbance (difficulty falling asleep, staying asleep, and early morning awakening) and decreased appetite (he had a 10-pound weight loss). There was an absence of "joie d' vie," which was replaced by a sense of human helplessness and knowledge of life's uncertainty and fragility. Carlos also reported having intense nightmares that affected his sleep. Prior to seeing me, he was placed on Lunesta, a sleep medication, by a colleague who prescribed it as a brief intervention.

Diagnosis: Post-Traumatic Stress Disorder 309.81 moderate to severe

Treatment

During our therapeutic conversations when Carlos described flashbacks of the accident, he often referred to conversations he had with Michele prior to the accident. These conversations, similar to a "living will," related to what each wanted the other to do if either of them were injured to the point of not being able to live life as vital human beings—whether to be heroic and try to save each other or to let the other die "in peace." There was a difficult-to-describe tone of "shock" in his voice as he repeatedly talked about his choices… and the "what ifs he had made a different decision at the moment." The tone of his voice conveyed intense fear, horror, and "astoundment." It is important to note that Carlos began his treatment with me during the time that although Michele was alive, we were unsure as to what her cognitive, emotional, and physical impairments would be….

Carlos and Michele are extraordinarily social people. Michele being Italian and Carlos, Portuguese, they construct their lives in the context of an extended family composed of people who are both biologically related and those who become "family" through friendship. With Michele in the hospital, their "family" stepped in to help Carlos. This cannot be minimized. In many ways, this was emotionally lifesaving. At the same time, part of Carlos's struggle was how to accept this support with appropriate boundaries and balance both his need to be taken care of and his need for autonomy.

[Process of Therapy description]

[signed] Dr. S., MD

As a psychiatrist, it was evident to Carlos that the relentless stress of this situation was taking a measurable toll upon him. He had frequent, disruptive nightmares. Although he was relatively uninjured aside from a bruised knee, he still had vivid memories of the event, even of pulling me off the fence where my head was wedged. While one might consider me lucky for not remembering the TBI incident, like other severe traumatic brain injury survivors, the same cannot be said for on-scene observers like Carlos, my mom, and my dad. It is possible that those with less severe TBIs who might not have as much brain trauma or loss of consciousness could also have harrowing memories of the event. As Dr. S reported, Carlos found himself startling at the sound of loud noises and pausing more than usual before crossing busy streets. His mind was remembering the details of the accident frequently.

Seeking treatment does not mean that this problem just goes away. Many years later, I still find Carlos unable or unwilling to relive this part of our lives. Carlos was agitated whenever I perseverated on the details I was trying to recapture about the lost time in my memory. I admit that I dogged him with questions about timelines and responses. However, Carlos felt the need to place his thoughts elsewhere and move forward, which is a characteristic he maintains to this day. At the time, he knew that he was wrestling with unavoidable anxiety and his own post-traumatic stress symptoms, and it was a painful time he would not like to relive, ever.

The caregiver is the one who must endure the brunt of the patient, address the challenges they face in a loving and compassionate manner, and put their own needs second in the moment. Caregiving is an important albeit draining role to play in a loved one's life. Lee Woodruff channeled her thoughts and emotions about the recovery and caregiving process of Bob's TBI in the aforementioned book *In an Instant*. Undoubtedly, the act of writing was a form of therapy to reconcile what had happened with the future of caring for prominent journalists and news anchor Bob, likely for the rest of his life. Many years later, Lee continues to write books and do speaking engagements. In addition to starting a foundation to support survivors of brain injury, Bob himself recently appeared with his son in a travel series called *Rogue* on Disney+ (2020).

As Dr. S. observed, I was lucky to have a wide net of caregivers, cheerleaders, and sources of support. I had Carlos, Eric, my mom, my dad, Suzi, Ana, Helena, Cindy, and other friends and family visit and take turns assisting me while Carlos was working. This is to say nothing of the hired rehab therapists and specialists who also provided me with care. It was a job for a village, and while I acknowledge how much I wanted to be *over* with the process and go back to being independent, I want to thank everyone who showed up for (and put up with) me during those first several months. I would not be where I am today without you.

During this tumultuous period, from weeks 8 to 12 following the injury, quiet for us as a couple had been replaced by the few minutes each day that lingered in the frequent transitions between doctor and rehab appointments. The steady influx of rehabilitative caregivers left very little time to ascertain what was happening to the life we had painstakingly built for years. For Carlos, even the time he had for solitary reflection seemed overrun by phone calls, emails, visits, and the expectations of others in his new job or dealing with my recovery. This is also because we elected to have the specialists and caregivers to come to me at home, rather than be shuttled to a rehab facility, since I couldn't drive myself. I also despise waiting, so in-home care was the absolute best option for me.

On a stolen walk in our neighborhood one evening, away from anyone in our growing healthcare entourage, I turned to Carlos and said, "How are *you* doing with all of this?" The question took him aback. The reality of his stress was so intense that he grappled with what would be right to say. His first response was a tentative and slightly atypical, "I'm not sure."

The soulful questions that were haunting him then hovered in a space that is common for next-of-kin in the depths of the survivor's guilt. I had just faced the fight of my life and was now forced to relearn various aspects of practically everything I once knew. Even though Carlos had his health in spite of being in the same accident, he was finding himself completely ill-equipped to process what transformation was taking place in his relationship with his wife. My impatience with my circumstances and combativeness against Carlos as the enforcer of rules was twisting our relationship into a difficult shape. He was not sure what was happening to the woman he loved inside me. Had I lost affection for him as a result of the injury? What did loving me now require? What were his obligations to me? To what extent would he be expected to provide for me? If I was never able to return to life the way we had once structured it, was he supposed to dismantle all of it and make me his primary focus? What kind of life did either of us need or want now?

Carlos wrestled with his response. Back in April, while I was still in hospital at USC and barely able to talk, he had been seated in the office of the neurologist supervising my case and listened gravely as the colleague and friend displayed the films of my scans. Struggling with her own emotions, the neurologist stated that she had never seen such extreme bilateral concussive damage, as evident in my frontal lobe, to be compatible with returning to a professional career. Carlos had misgivings about what information like that would do to my determination to recover. Furthermore, he had already seen me exceed so many of the prognostic expectations since the ordeal began. Therefore, on the walk in May, he offered me the belief that he had arrived at: "Michele, no one truly knows what you are going to be able to get back to." I then told Carlos that we both still had a lot of work to do. I admitted that if I was standing in his shoes, I would give it about a year to see how recovery would take shape.

It is also important to mention that primary caregivers are not always partners or spouses. Sometimes parents, siblings, children, or close friends step in to assume the role. Claudia Osborne, author of *Over My Head*, a memoir about her own TBI and subsequent recovery through the NYU brain injury program, relied heavily on her roommate for support.

Society uses the term "self-care" to refer to how much attention we pay to our own health (mental and physical). This is especially true for caregivers, who put others' needs above theirs all the time. Caregivers also require the help of friends, family, professionals, or support groups. Although it is said that it is better to give than receive, it is also better to ask for help than to struggle in silence. Regardless, caregivers are the lynchpin to any TBI patient's recovery.

Legs

11

Everything should be made as simple as possible, but not simpler.

—Albert Einstein, physicist

I was always looking outside myself for strength and confidence, but it comes from within. It is there all the time.

—Anna Freud, psychoanalyst

As best I could, I continued to make progress in my recovery. Carlos was working harder than ever, and the duties were more elaborate than in jobs past. The constant concerns for me were two things: I wished I could run and work like I used to before the accident. Nothing could come soon enough. And then there was the dynamic between Carlos and me, or the issue of "us": I wanted to carry equal weight in the relationship too.

What I never realized (how could I have?) was how my brain injury made an immediate impact on and even inspired others. Sean Linehan, Eric's best friend, wrote his high school senior paper about my injury. Although that report has since been lost due to the passage of time and obsolete technology, we remember that Sean came out to California to visit us with his parents, Jim and Pat (friends that we refer to as our "family by friendship"), and witnessed my early recovery firsthand. Clearly, my accident had profound ripple effects across the many people in my life.

Luckily, I was able to fly to DC to attend Eric's high school graduation at Walt Whitman High in June. This again was our choice. The doctors thought it was too early, but Carlos supported my belief that it was good for my mental health. He coined the phrase, "We should refuse to be prisoners of your prognosis." Since we had just sold our house in Bethesda, we stayed in a hotel for the ceremony. Carlos and I were so proud of Eric and felt extremely grateful for his decision to be with

M. T. Pato, *Nerve*, https://doi.org/10.1007/978-3-031-33433-7_11

me after the accident. Despite all the upheaval in his life, he was succeeding and
moving on to the next chapter in his life (Fig. 11.1).

After graduation, Eric visited and stayed with his aunt (and godmother), Carlos's
sister Ana, in Syracuse for a week with her family, from June 13th to 20th. All things
considered, he was doing well and expressed to them that he was very excited about
attending New York University Film School in the fall. He explained that I was
improving steadily and showing fewer symptoms but that the whole situation was still
emotionally draining. It was pleasant for him also to be around his grandparents (my
in-laws) and his old friends from Syracuse and try to regain some sense of normalcy.
About me, he remarked that I couldn't "stay up and run with the wild ones anymore,"
which was figuratively and literally true. Resting was a necessity to be able to function
at all. It was an adjustment, and not just because of my own restless legs!

I learned a long time ago, perhaps when I was playing soccer at 17, that I do best
when both my body and brain are in motion. In my adulthood, I have looked forward to deliberately putting a thought in my head and then heading out the door for
a run. As my legs pound the ground and my arms swing through the air, I won't
belabor the thought, letting it just flow back and forth in the back of my brain.

Scientific studies show that imprinting memories and overall cognition are
boosted after a physical activity such as running. This is to say nothing of the eupho-
ria that your body can experience from the physical accomplishment of building
such endurance. As a doctor myself, I know that the human body generates endor-
phins and enkephalins with this kind of exertion, and there's no denying that most
people know when something is satisfying and just "feels good."

Repeating the same motion or task also creates neuromuscular memories. Play
the same eight bars of a piano piece over and over until you stop thinking about it,
and you'll find your fingers almost move on their own, just where you want. Cut and
form several batches of snickerdoodles, then roll them in cinnamon and sugar, and
you'll end up with four dozen cookies that look and taste the same in 8–10 min.
Believe it or not, these repetitive behaviors help you solve problems you are stuck

Fig. 11.1 First plane
flight, back east, for son's
high school graduation

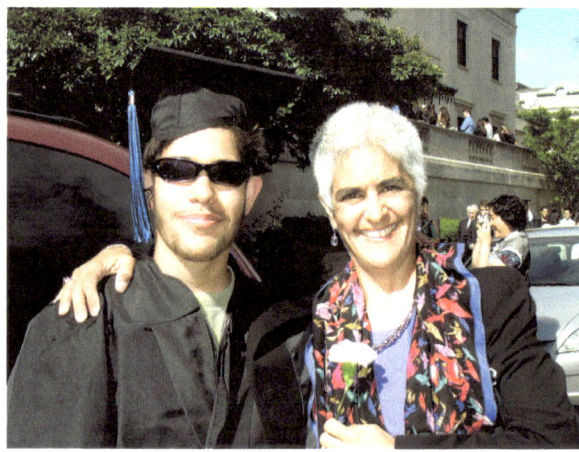

on. When new things are creating obstacles, it is comforting to return to something you know you can do. Quite simply, running clears my head. When my brain is stumped, and it sure was during this point in my recovery, running seemed like the answer to all my worries.

Upon returning to work that summer with rather short hair, I came into contact with a number of my new co-faculty. Most had heard about my accident, but few had truly known me before the TBI, since I had only been officially employed at USC for a month (I started on March 1, 2006). Consistently, the reaction was, "Oh my god! You are alive! And talking!" However, within a month or two, my hair grew back to my normal length, which was still short overall. Now that the 6–8 in. scar on my scalp was covered by hair, my injury had been largely forgotten. Or rather, it seemed that way, until 1 day, when Carlos received an email from a senior faculty colleague whom I had written a report for. He was wondering in light of a recent document that he had gotten from me if this poor quality was always how I wrote! Carlos thought for a moment and said, "Oh, is it a first draft?" The faculty member responded that yes it was.

Eventually Carlos came back to me with this story and said, "Michele, remember the people here don't know you. I read your first drafts all the time, and I know you just like to get ideas down; that's why you ask me to edit them. Why didn't you do that this time?" To which I said, "Well, I didn't want to burden you even more. I know how much you have had to fill in since my TBI." He explained to me that if we always did this before, then we should continue to do it now. My style was to take down all, and sometimes too many, facts and details, without concern about spelling or grammar. This is what makes Carlos and I such a good research and writing team. I'm the raw data/information gatherer and he's the polished wordsmith. It was a powerful lesson. You shouldn't have to get rid of ingrained behaviors and strategies that worked for you before the injury. With change, look back to the familiar.

By July, 3 months after the accident, we began planning for a trip to Portugal for Carlos to receive an honorary doctorate in a ceremony at University of Coimbra. On the way, we would make a stop in Boston to rest in between those 6-h flights and combat jetlag. Although I had been on a few flights across coasts before, getting my bearings with a longer, cross-ocean flight was a concern. Additionally, at this point, I was desperately trying to reintegrate into my new position at USC. I was greeted by colleagues with a reaction that most were impressed that I was alive and could walk and talk. Although that was somewhat insulting to me, in hindsight I could see that it was a human response upon hearing what had happened. Sure, it was a miraculous recovery and return to work, but as a patient, I could only see what I had lost, not what I had regained.

By the time we left for Portugal on July 15th, I was cleared and back to running again. This had been so important to me, to regain this part of my routine. In the past, the average day even before my TBI, starting in medical school at age 23, began at 6 a.m. The first hour I dedicated to strength training. Once completed, I replied to the morning's flood of emails before setting out on my daily 30-min, 2- to 3-mile run. To be able to put running back into my life was huge; many family members thought this was the missing puzzle piece in my ability to make a near-complete recovery. If I could get my legs under me and run, all things would flow more easily from there.

The ceremony in Portugal was huge and filled with friends and family. It was such a big deal for Carlos to receive this honor and for me to be able to attend. Those 2 weeks were magical for us. We were greeted and recognized by family, friends, and colleagues who had known us as a couple who were also researchers and doctors since before we were even married. It was back in 1979 that I made my first trip abroad, with my first passport, with Carlos. When he was 7, Carlos and his immediate family moved to the United States from Portugal. I remember practicing my newly learned language by announcing our engagement to many in Carlos's family in Portuguese. Without even knowing it, I was a big success! This was significant because other non-Portuguese-speaking spouses who had married into the family did not try to learn or speak the language. However, for me I couldn't imagine not being able to communicate for myself, and not having the understanding of another culture that would be so much a part of my life. Although as is traditional for many Portuguese families, Carlos returned, almost yearly, to visit "home," and we would continue to do so after our marriage. I love the word in Portuguese that captures this "longing" for home, *saudade*. It's more than simply homesickness. It's truly more a term of respect for wanting to spend time in a place that is also part of who you are (Fig. 11.2).

Fig. 11.2 Return again to Portugal with family and friends for Carlos' honorary doctorate

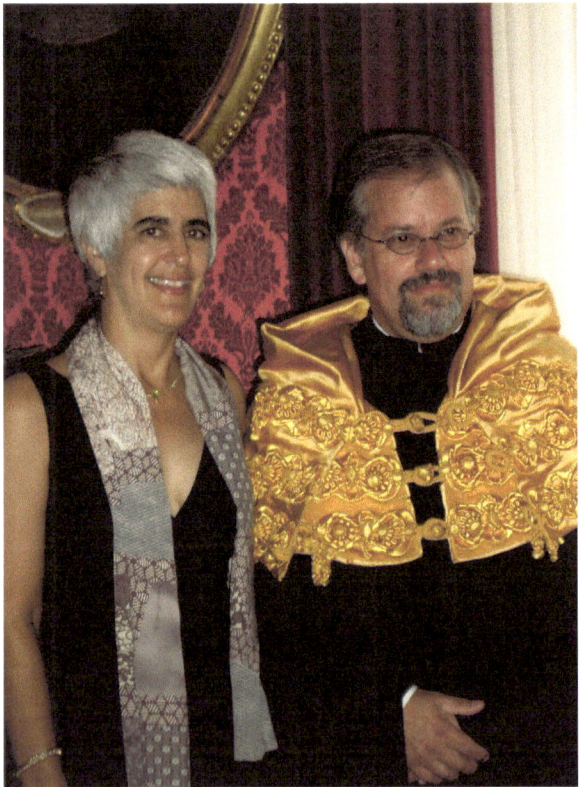

In our 40 years of marriage, I have been to Portugal more than 45 times. So this return in our 26th year of marriage was surely familiar, and with people who had known me a long time, and had also learned long distance of my TBI. This was a much more familiar and comforting experience than meeting new colleagues and friends at USC just a few weeks before, for they had not "known" me before my injury. Not only did my adopted Portuguese family recognize me, but they calmed any apprehension I had about being the same as I was before my injury. While a number of them were doctors themselves, and thus very worried about my recovery, they marveled at my recovery. Their encouragement was genuine and rooted in 26 years of history. Therefore, in addition to the celebrations for Carlos's honorary doctorate, this was a real time of grounding and celebration for me. I could feel I was getting myself back.

It was in Portugal when I finally got my legs firmly under me and ran as I always had before. It was unusual for a girl to run on the sidewalks in Portugal. This is despite the country's most famous female runner, Rosa Mota, who won several marathons and the Seoul Olympics in 1988. Although Lisbon and Coimbra were modern and academic cities, few women ran the streets. With my dark Italian hair and olive skin, I fit in as southern European, but I was still noticeable. However, I didn't mind sticking out. I was used to it. In the farming countryside of Mamarrosa, I was even more of a female oddity, running on the pavementless dirt streets and grass soccer (*futbol* in Portuguese) fields. Running had always made me get to know the neighborhoods better, and I found the right pace to pay attention to my surroundings while still going fast. This time I felt everything as familiar and being at home, *saudade*.

Ligament

12

A person's life may be a lonely thing by nature, but it is not isolated. To that life other lives are linked.

—Haruki Murakami, author

Character cannot be developed in ease and quiet. Only through experience of trial and suffering can the soul be strengthened, ambition inspired, and success achieved.

—Helen Keller, author and activist

After our trip to Portugal, life seemed to move on at an alarming clip. That is, we moved on as a family in the only way we knew how: *Avanti*! Forward! In asking my husband and sons what happened that fall, Christmas, or New Year following the accident, like me, they don't remember much. Both boys were away at college, Carlos was continuing his work tirelessly, and I was settling in, to my own rhythm, at USC. My hair grew back furiously, and many new people I worked with had no idea what I had been through. This was no help, however, in my struggle to remember their names. In addition, those who were aware of the circumstances, outside of being supportive of my "miraculous" recovery, showed a bit of tenuousness that I was previously unaccustomed to: would I be able to function? To teach? To excel? (Figs. 12.1 and 12.2).

This mistrust, which I now take as a natural reaction to someone who had half her skull removed months earlier, was unsettling at the time. I've established that my personality is one that "takes no prisoners" and forges a path toward any goal and gets there. In addition, although I needed to overcome some initial deficits, which I will go into more detail about later, my drive and determination remained the same. This was just a bump in the road for me. For others in my professional life, it was a serious question. Doubt is a four-letter word if you know what I mean. So I pressed forward.

Fig. 12.1 Visit the old haunts in Newport, RI, with sons Mike and Eric just 4 months after bone is back

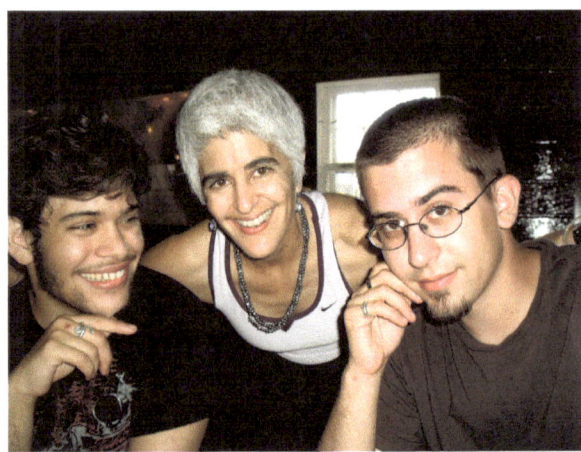

Fig. 12.2 Connecting with "the Girls," in California, who were always rooting for my recovery

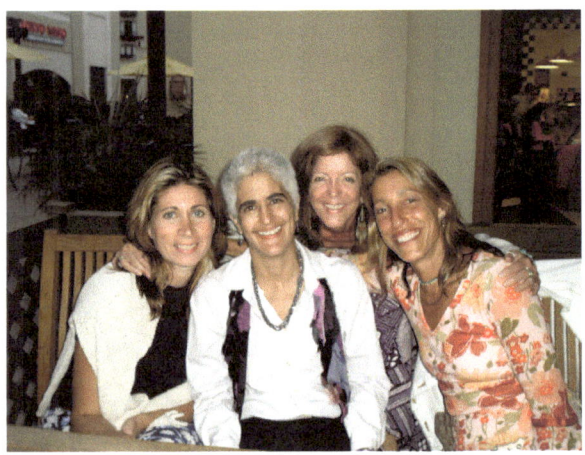

If 2006 was punctuated sharply by the accident, 2007 was remarkable because my father, Tony Tortora, at 75 years old, received a leiomyosarcoma diagnosis, which is a type of cancer that affects the lungs. At the time of his first appointment in January 2007, at Memorial Sloan Kettering Cancer Center, which Suzi helped to orchestrate, he was given only 6 months to live. However, he continued to work as an engineer. As a Tortora, and any Italian, you basically worked until the day you died, just like your/his parents. There was no way that he wanted to stop working while receiving treatment, so to continue to go to job sites and inspect the air-conditioning and heating contracts, he refrained from using an oxygen tank. At the end of June 2008, almost 18 months later, he began to receive oxygen through a face mask. Nevertheless, he studied drafts of buildings they were working on on a large drafting table in his home. Once he suffered another episode of extreme shortness of breath in late July or early August, he insisted upon going into a hospice and made himself a DNR (Do Not Resuscitate) order. Both of these decisions were not made lightly. He and I had long, matter-of-fact conversations that perhaps he couldn't have with my mother or sister, who are more outwardly sensitive and empathic people. When it came to such scientific data, we could connect! One night after he had just been released from the hospital to his home in Garrison, NY, he ended up sleeping on the first-floor sofa since he could no longer climb stairs with his shortness of breath. It hadn't occurred to my parents to rent a hospital bed, as they had always slept together in the bed in their bedroom upstairs. Therefore, the next day we moved furniture around to accommodate the delivery of a hospital bed on the main floor. Two days later, after we had all welcomed him home and left, the power went out in the middle of the night. In the dark, my mother came "running" literally down the stairs with a flashlight, panicked because he was experiencing shortness of breath again. She called me later that morning to tell me what had happened, and Suzi and I both insisted that she take him back to the hospital where he could be better taken care of, knowing that he would request the hospice once he got to the hospital. Although this came as a great shock to her, I wasn't surprised that he didn't want to die at home. He wanted my mother to stay there after he passed (where she still is after 10+ years) and didn't want his death to be a memory locked into that place. Rather, he preferred that my mom and the rest of the family would have the home as a reminder of the joys of their life together. Therefore, he and I agreed that going into a hospice would be better.

It was around this time that I began contemplating how his death would change or impact the family. I didn't want to rush such crucial conversations, but I did want to have a talk with my sons about life and loss. This was the first grandparent, in fact the only one, to die thus far; such grief would be unfamiliar to them. In addition, although my dad's illness was 18 months long, he had been very healthy beforehand, so there had been little preparation for the severity and relatively rapid progression of it. Great grandparents had passed but only after chronic, protracted cancer battles and Alzheimer's. As I recount this, I am struck by the similarities to TBI. By its very definition, TBI is something sudden and unplanned just like the aggressive and fast-growing cancer, leiomyosarcoma, my dad had. With modern medicine, many of those who survive the initial trauma of TBI must still be prepared for disability (if not death in the future). Tough end-of-life discussions and decisions come to the forefront, just as with any other difficult or terminal diagnosis. Just the year before both boys had experienced the near-death experience of me their mother and neither had truly talked about it much since. Grandpa's, my dad's, imminent death appeared to be an opportunity to begin to prepare them for the natural course of any life which includes death. It also gave me a chance to talk to them about things that I could still recall and remember around my own near-death experience. Memory loss can come earlier for those with TBI even when it is not simply in the time around the injury (retrograde and antegrade amnesia) and kind of like my dad I wanted to communicate while I could still. We talked about plans after college, about getting married, about what it meant to have a spouse and a family, and about how they might want to pass on parts of our shared history, like the yearly trips to the family home in Portugal, family ski trips, and surviving my TBI. Once you have had a TBI, there are always the thoughts of "shoulda, coulda, woulda," and here was an opportunity to avoid that.

Even though we had multiple signed copies of the DNR, dad and I both felt that mom might not be able to follow through on it and would call an ambulance and let them resuscitate him. Therefore, the added benefit of being in a hospice is that they would follow through on his DNR requests to not intubate or resuscitate with CPR or electroconversion. I said, "Dad, no one in our family dies of heart attacks, it's usually cancer. Our hearts are pretty healthy. Therefore, when your heart stops beating, it is going to be because of your lung cancer, the heart muscle isn't getting enough oxygen." Then, I said, "And what other organ do you think won't be getting oxygen besides your heart?" He paused only a minute and looked at me and said, "My brain. Let's do a full DNR and get me to a hospice when there is no hope. I don't want a tube down my throat to breathe and I don't want to be brain dead and still breathing. I'm old and I've had a good life up until now, and if I can't even talk, why do I need to live longer? Will it even be living if I can't tell you what I'm thinking?" These had been my thoughts exactly!

I have come to realize that for all of us Tortoras, and maybe my mom's Rosset side as well, nothing is more important to us than the brain. You can push the physical body to its limits and compensate. My mom's sister, Anita, survived polio with a limp and had three kids when the doctor told her to stop at two. My father's mother, Nana, made her final Seven Fishes Christmas dinner on December 24, 1985, when I was 5 months' pregnant with Michael, who would have been her first great grandchild, and died the same day they planned her retirement party at Bloomingdale's in January of 1986. In addition, so it was with my dad, I think he died in the hospice with floor plans draped over his body in bed. He would remove the oxygen mask because the flow rate was so high and noisy, so he could speak to us, even though his throat was incredibly dry. He still had more things to say. I only found out recently from Suzi, that in that first week in hospice as his illness progressed, he confided in her that he was worried that dying would feel like drowning. My sister reached out to colleagues at Memorial Sloan Kettering Cancer Center, who reassured her that he would go into coma and not experience that sensation. When she told him this, he was relieved and within 48 h, he passed away peacefully.

We had a simple prayer service with his ashes on Saturday, August 23rd, at 10:30 a.m. just for the immediate family. No big Italian funeral with a long procession and lots of crying and drinking; he made it very clear he did not want that. Instead, we had a "Celebration of Life" gathering with upward of 50 family and friends. We asked people to share any memories from childhood to recent vacations they had been on with my dad and mom. It was a tearful and joyous event to recall our memories together. I also shared a quote sometimes attributed to George Carlin: "Life is not measured by the number of breaths you take, but by the moments that take your breath away." I told the story of how I changed my major for the fourth time during my senior year when I was home again for Christmas from college. This time, I was again changing my major and applying to medical school. To which dad replied with a laugh and smile, "Finally, it's what I always wanted for you but I know you had to decide for yourself." That was my dad! Do what you want, but do it with passion and love it for what it is.

Looking back, he was just ten paces behind me walking with my mother on the same sidewalk in Pittsburgh. He watched the car hit me, left my mother on the sidewalk near where Carlos found me, and went right to the scene of the accident to help control the elderly man who was too confused to comprehend what he had just done. While standing there with this man, he called my sister back home in New York, telling her that I had been hit by a car and very badly injured. My sister was on a plane within 4 h. My dad was always a doer and a fixer that he would help you do things, but in the tone of his voice, she was sensing, for the first time, that he needed her help too, which was very rare. In fact, as he faced his own death just 2 years later, our discussion was much more a deliberation between two colleagues than a matter of asking for help, as was Suzi's about not having to have a fear that he would feel like he was drowning when he passed.

In writing this book, my sister, Suzi, also recently revealed to me that when I was in coma, he had told her that he was not sure if he could go on living if I died. My own interpretation of that, although I am not sure if it would be hers, was he was saying that the things we shared in common and the way we could talk and understand each other would be so missed. If I were gone, his will to live would wither. This may be one reason why I'm so compelled to write about how important family and friends can be in TBI recovery. Sometimes the help from family and friends will vary at different points of your recovery. Or you may need the help of different family members or friends at different times.

It was so "Tortora" to just add things and not stop doing anything no matter what the crisis. Suzi, having been by his side until the end, left for a trip for her work to Argentina on August 25th just 2 days after the brief church service. It had been his wish that she continue her work, her worldwide trips spreading her work in dance therapy around the world, no matter what his physical condition. Even after his death, Eric, who was no longer a practicing churchgoer, would not come in for the ceremony. He said he was going to stay outside the church "with grandpa," who was not much of a churchgoer himself, except to come to my wedding in 1980 and lead me down the aisle. My mother had plans of her own, including a photography trip to Iceland, a once-in-a-lifetime experience that my father made me promise that she would follow through on and she did.

I often talk about how I am cut from two cloths: an engineer and an artist. My methodical, logical side comes from my father, and my mother has always had a passion for art. She took her first photography class in 1974, the same year I graduated high school, and went on to pursue a master's degree in photography from Long Island University thereafter. She describes her discovery of photography as a vocation like this: "I realized that I had been seeing the world through a camera all my life. I had been constantly framing whatever was in front of me. In addition, the first time I put a piece of photo paper into chemicals, watching as an image I made emerged I could not believe the magic that was taking place! The very reason photography appeals to me is its ability to capture what I see. Words have always been difficult for me, seeing has always been easy but until I found photography, images flew through my mind, never caught. Beauty is a fragile ingredient in life, fleeing quickly. Being able to capture one moment is a treasure. I view this capturing as a never-ending process that fills my need to communicate with others." My father built her a darkroom, and she developed her talent using the Holga camera and creative layering techniques. Although showing little interest in the sale of her work, my mother thrives in this medium still and has garnered excellent reviews from the *New York Times* and other noteworthy newspapers.

When an opportunity arose in late 2007 to showcase my mother's work at the USC's Institute for Genetic Medicine Art Gallery, I jumped at the chance to support her and connected her to the director of the gallery. As it happened, the show took place in November 2008 after dad's death in August. He had made me promise to make the show happen whether he could be there or not. The exhibition, titled "Transformation: Capturing the Moment," combined the elements of fragmentation, layering, black/white, positive and negative space, and a "career-long exploration of Urban Order and Destruction, Bridges and Walk-ways, and The Force of Nature":

[ARTIST'S STATEMENT] (Fig. 12.3)

Transformation: Capturing the Moment

Fragmentation, along with the interplay of positive and negative space as it relates to form, is the element of my photographs. Black and white and the shades in between comprise my world of color. I am drawn to the beauty in the world that surrounds me both manmade and natural. Buildings, canyons, and landscapes each become part of a reconstructed image. These transformations are inspired by the cubist concept of revealing an object from different points of view. To create my photographs, I often cut my contact sheets and reassemble them to make a new image that flows. While interested in the individual photographs, it is their reconstruction that I focus on. My hope is to communicate the beauty I see around me through these transformations.

I longed to arrest all beauty that came before me, and at length the longing has been satisfied. This quote by Julia Margaret Cameron closely expresses my feelings, explaining the very reason I think photography so appealed to me. I "see" the beauty in all the views around me. To be able to capture this beauty that I thought I could only see for myself and to give it to others is the joy I find in this very expressive art form. I no longer have to say, "Look at this! Isn't it wonderful; please pay attention to the beauty around you." I now only have to capture the moment. Words have always been difficult; seeing has always been easy, but until I found photography, images flew through my mind, never caught. The longing has been satisfied, the images remain, hopefully others will "see" the way I see, enjoy my images as I do and feel a moment of contentment.

Beauty, a very fragile ingredient of life, is quick to flee. Capturing one moment is a treasure. I see this capturing as a never-ending process that fills my need to communicate with others. To quote Martha Graham, *However, art is eternal: for it reveals the inner landscape which is the soul of man.*

—Lucille Tortora

The debut of this exhibition was on November 6, 2008, just over 2 months after my father had passed. I delivered the keynote address—*"All Our Life Experiences Are Connected:* Decision-Making and Risk-Taking in Uncertain Times." The goal was to show the connection between art and mental and physical health and whether it helped maintain your well-being (or aid with recovery). Perhaps for my mom and I, this was a chance to do both. I suspect this brought focus on her still needing to

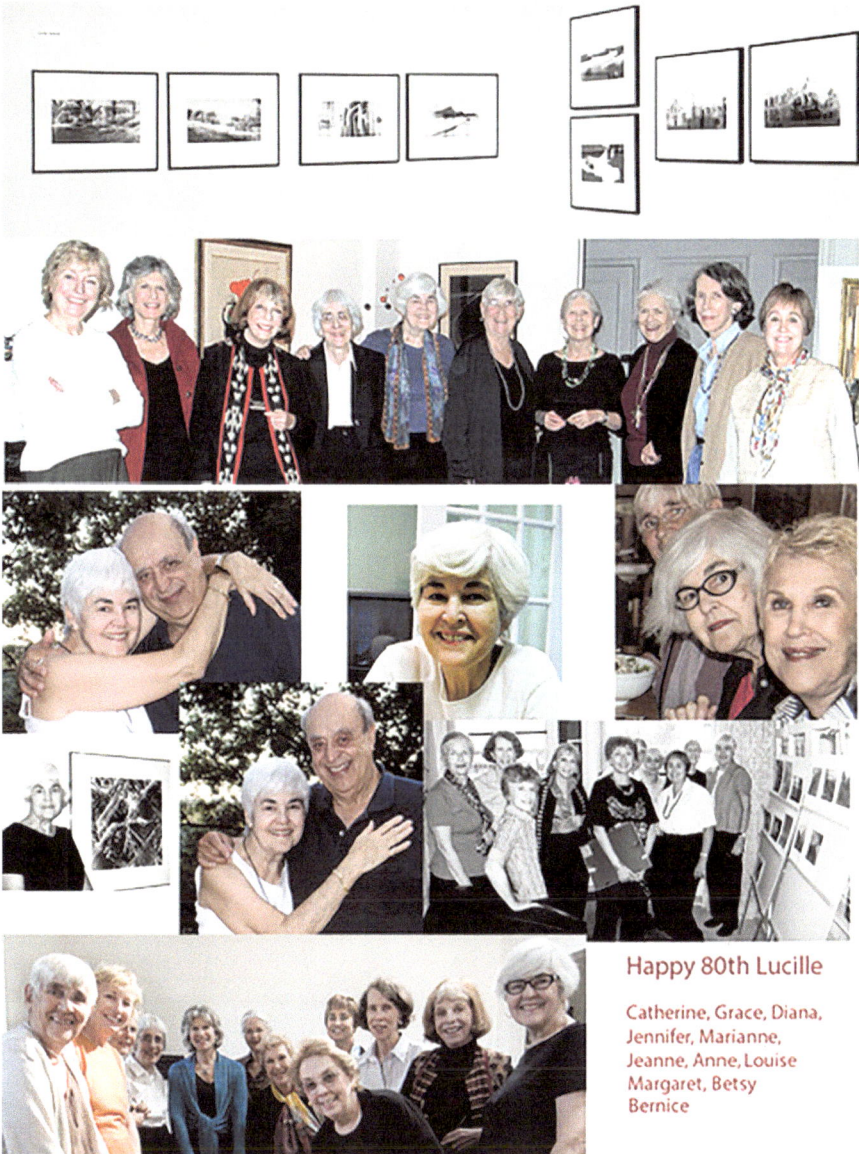

Happy 80th Lucille

Catherine, Grace, Diana,
Jennifer, Marianne,
Jeanne, Anne, Louise
Margaret, Betsy
Bernice

Fig. 12.3 Friends and family kept my mom (in the purple shirt) and dad going as well. Here's some of the work in her show in 2008 as well

recover emotionally from my injury, which was only 2 years before, and in the end I think it helped her deal with the loss of her husband as well. As my father was dying in July and August, he made sure to say many times in our conversations in front of Mom that even if he couldn't get to the show out in California, we should still make sure to have it. For me, it was a chance to take stock of what TBI had taught me as well as what I had learned being the child of an engineer and an artist.

That June and July, my mom thought of backing out of her trip to Iceland that was scheduled for November 2nd, because she didn't want to be away when dad died, although I wonder, if he had lived that long, might he have been relieved that she was away? My mother did go to Iceland on the second, which meant that she wasn't present at the opening of her own show on the 6th! I delivered the keynote to a crowd of 40–60 people, and the show ran for approximately 2 months. It was nice in a way to talk to a room of strangers, people who just came to see the show because they were drawn to the art, by then it was also slightly more apparent how art can inform life experiences like loss or near loss of a loved one. Death and near-death experiences (NDE) such as mine are hard for anyone to face, although perhaps we do not focus enough on the surviving family members after a loved one's death or NDE. TBI was a near-death experience for me. Maybe supporting and helping me through it was a way for my family and friends to cope with the traumatic experience themselves.

Just as the art exhibition demonstrated the connections between man and nature and our emotional and scientific worlds, it also highlights the connections between us and how much we rely on each other. Without my father, my mother would never have had the courage to pursue photography. Without my family, I would never have survived TBI. Adversity, and even loss or the threat of loss, profoundly strengthens our ties, our connections, the ligament between us. When one muscle or tendon is weak, another adjacent muscle or tendon is leaned upon to bear the load.

Backbone

13

A tree trunk the size of a man grows from a blade as thin as a hair. A tower nine stories high is built from a small heap of earth.

—Lao Tzu, philosopher

The tree is more than first a seed, then a stem, then a living trunk, and then dead timber. The tree is a slow, enduring force straining to win the sky.

—Antoine de Saint-Exupery, author

Overall, I can attest that the experience of recovering from TBI dragged on and flew by all at once. When I look back especially on the first 4 years of my recovery, there were moments when my progress felt like it was moving at a snail's pace. For some people, the past can haunt you. It forces you to confront your newfound deficits, and you could easily become trapped by negative thinking and setbacks. However, the past can also propel you forward, as it did for me. When I realized what I had lost, I also began to appreciate what I had "kept" and learned how I could use those skills to regain my physical senses (if possible) and remediate my capacity to communicate. When I began the journey back to normal life, my typing, speech, and malapropisms were at approximately 75% versus the 95% they are today. Life became more about repurposing rather than returning exactly as I once was.

However, with my Just Do It™ Nike-like attitude, unchanged from before my injury, I wanted to jump into everything at once: reclaim my family life, my social life, and my academic career. However, trees grow slowly, and when you knock off or cut down branches, they require time, and patience, to regenerate and sometimes grow in ways that they hadn't before. Therefore, I had to build my backbone, like the trunk of a tree, so to speak.

You've read a lot already about how my family and friends helped me. I hosted small dinner parties with one or two couples at a time to thank my friends and

M. T. Pato, *Nerve*, https://doi.org/10.1007/978-3-031-33433-7_13

family for their support. I also did this to prove that I could still cook, albeit it was a messier and more accident-prone experience. Unable to smell, I easily burned and threw out more food than usual. I never seemed to know if milk had gone sour until it ended up curdled when combined with coffee or tea, so it became a habit some mornings to bring the gallon to Carlos in bed and ask him, "Is this milk bad?" No one complained about my cooking or small foibles, although, and so it appeared that maybe I was just being my own stern judge. Even when I was frustrated with the process, I was more than happy to be talking and interacting with people I loved and respected again.

The road to my academic recovery, by contrast, was a lot harder. For one thing, my tenure at USC was still in its infancy since my injury happened only 1 month after officially starting my job there. The overall reaction was astonishment that I had survived and then chose to come back. It was lucky that I still had connections to my previous jobs and organizations that I had belonged to for 10–20 years to fall back on. These were all the people who "knew" me before my injury and could remember what I was capable of. It made the most sense to tap into some of these resources to help reestablish my academic reputation.

As much as I relied on what and who I knew, there were some new connections that I was able to make after my recovery in those early years. My friend and future colleague Cynthia Harrington and I met at my mother's photography exhibition. She was interested in my keynote about transformation in behavioral science because she came from a behavioral finance background. The next week, Cynthia joined us, along with USC's chair of internal medicine and his wife, in the Little Tokyo neighborhood for sushi. We hit it off and began spending holidays and other occasions together. When the financial crisis of 2008 had broken the market, Cynthia got out of the sector. Sharing a mutual interest in healing and therapy, we began collaborating on projects for the CFA Society of Los Angeles, stress management, coaching pension fund managers, and integrative software for teachers.

She recalls, "Throughout all this time, when I met Michele and when I met other people along with her, the story of the accident came up within the first few hours. She explained that there was something to be aware of with her, something to watch for or to allow for because she was different. In addition, in all of these—100 percent of these conversations—I brushed it off. It was clear to me that the dynamic, articulate, brilliant, energetic woman that I knew may have had a profound experience with this accident. However, to any observer, it had not negatively impacted her life. She was bothered by it although and needed everyone she knew to share in this knowledge that something had happened that was deep and profound."

It occurs to me that I disclosed my injury so soon after meeting new people because I felt a great need to get it out of the way. While old friends understood, new friends, I had determined, should be warned. Rather than having an issue crop up later regarding my injury and recent recovery, I wanted that caveat out front.

Cynthia also remembered one evening later in our relationship:

We met a lead scientist on Michele and Carlos's team, Jim Knowles. We sat at a long table, with many other members of the team who I had met on several occasions, and at some point the conversation took a different turn. Carlos asked Michele, 'Do you think you are capable of handling that?' My stomach flipped. Could all of our work be for naught because she could not be counted on when time to present it? This was a private moment, one in which they shared a doubt of her competency. I thought of all the work we were doing together in this moment of doubt and wondered at my own powers of observation. How could we be doing this high level of educated and creative work and she be at any, even small, level of disability? After that, I tried to observe her carefully, yet I still saw no difference. Years later, I concluded that maybe both their private doubt and my observations of public presentations were correct. Here is a person with so much talent and intelligence that she could give up some and still be brilliant and capable.

Cynthia, an incredibly perceptive person, has helped me understand that the short-term challenge of my TBI did not substantially matter to people. What I was in that moment was good enough, no matter how much I struggled or felt the need to compensate.

Then, there were those situations that weren't new: organizations where I had known people for years and saw them at national meetings where I would often lead a symposium. For AADPRT, the organization for residency training directors in psychiatry, I received a premeeting grant for 5 years and did the first presentation, ironically in March 2006, not even 4 weeks before my accident. In March 2006, I had run my first year of the R-13 grant on teaching teachers how to teach. I went back and ran the second year of the grant in March 2007 and received a standing ovation after training director Grace Thrall introduced my return to the meeting just 11 months after my accident and TBI. All together I was involved in doing this R-13 for 10 years: 5 years as the PI (2006–2010) and then 5 years as the consultant (2011–2015).

I also remember having to be especially patient and work hard to move up in the ranks at the AAP, the association for teachers of psychiatry (Association for Academic Psychiatry) during this time. Previously, I had served as program director, and usually the protocol went that then you became treasurer, secretary, and finally president (if you still wanted the position). However, I did not go through the traditional moves from treasurer to secretary to president when I finished my term as program chair. I suspect that because my injury was April first, I missed the September meeting in 2006. I remember truly wanting to land the position of president as a way of proving I had in fact recovered.

In September 2007, just 18 months after my injury, I was awarded their education award and gave a keynote speech titled, "What to Learn and How to Teach It – The Efficacy and Effectiveness Literature." Perhaps that was the first proof for me and affirmed my competency and ability for the members of the organization too. Finally, in 2009, the AAP named me the president for 2010. Cynthia Harrington also came to this AAP talk in 2010. Some of the themes from the presidential presentation in September 2010 in Pasadena were as follows:

LifeLong Learning: Living in the Moment, Learning from the Past, and Looking to the Future truly helped me recover from my traumatic brain injury. I wasn't supposed to live and then I wasn't supposed to talk or walk again. In addition, no one even mentioned me returning to work; not my friends, my students, my colleagues, and my patients. However, no one told me what was *supposed* to happen so I did what I always did as a student, which was try to learn! I lived in the moment and took the challenge of what was facing me. My mother, who kept vigil at my bedside as I was in coma, was assured that when I sang and hummed "Amazing Grace" that she could look to the future, because what was once lost could be found.

Another quotation I love to use is "The best way to learn something is to teach it to someone else." Therefore, teaching others "to learn how to learn" is something I champion. For example, when I began typing again on my computer, I didn't want to slow down my speed too much because my keystroke rhythm was still there. However, then I did have to check more for typos, because my accuracy was definitely not what it used to be! This was and still can be exasperating. I recognize that there are some things that require an extra step or two to complete. I turn to the wisdom of others for reassurance, such as Sackett (1995): "Evidence-based medicine is not 'cookbook' medicine. Because it requires a bottom-up approach that integrates the best external evidence with individual clinical expertise and patients' choice, it cannot result in slavish, cookbook approaches to individual patient care." I often turn back to my most basic learning experiences, what grandma "Nana" taught me about cooking. When you are making a good tomato sauce, a ragu, you have to stir the bottom up to the top. You can't just let everything settle; you have to "stir it up." Sometimes I remember this concept and turn things on their head by reapproaching a problem in a new way.

Deliberate practice is necessary for the maintenance of any skill. Therefore, I had to go back to things that were familiar and then prove I knew them in order to determine what I had to learn as "new" again. What, in my career, might be holding me back, and what could I use to move forward? Therefore, I wondered, how can we offer ways of teaching and learning that are not automatic and lead to plateaus but rather offer paths to continued improvement?

The predominant themes in my keynotes and talks became centered around the concept of resilience: "a dynamic process encompassing positive adaptation within the context of significant adversity" (Luthar 2000b from Graham paper 2013). Moving forward with what you have despite severe challenge and adversity is what bouncing back is all about. Although my accident was a true test of my mettle, it put my own teachings into perspective. While the journey wasn't as quick or uncomplicated as I had hoped, I managed to regain my standing in the academic community in spite of the injuries. Perhaps I am now more focused and driven than ever.

Concurrently with my fight to prove myself at work, we decided to pursue a lawsuit against the city of Pittsburgh and the motorists involved in the accident. I'm not sure when it commenced exactly, but it continued on through 2008 and 2009. My reasons for pursuing this were to motivate the city to improve the intersection and to address the risk of driving once a person's capacity to do it safely has become limited. For the purposes of establishing the extent of my injuries, I underwent neurocognitive testing to determine my deficits, injuries, and compensations I had made cognitively as a result of the accident.

A series of examinations by Dr. W, a specialist in hearing, balance, and ear disorders, was performed and summarized on April 20, 2009, over 3 years after my injury. He provided a detailed written neuro-otology evaluation that detailed my complaints of hearing loss, tinnitus, vertigo and dysequilibrium, and headaches. This was an exhaustive evaluation aimed at pinpointing my deficits for the purposes of creating a record of my injury and identifying concrete damages caused by the accident. After presenting raw data, the following conclusions can be drawn:

Michele has had difficulty hearing since the injury (4/01/2006). She especially has problems with hearing in complex auditory environments (i.e., student voices in lecture halls). She always has increased awareness of any background noise. Increased background noise significantly affects her ability to hear. She noticed that her hearing sensitivity fluctuated throughout the day. Since the injury, she has noticed problems with fluctuant ear pressure (fullness) during airline travel. She has had bilateral tinnitus, right>>left, since the injury (4/1/2006). Tinnitus is described as an ocean like static-like sound. Tinnitus is always present. The tinnitus is bothersome. Tinnitus is most noticeable in quiet environments. Loudness of tinnitus in quiet can cause problems with concentration. She can forget things that she is told. She always uses her iPhone calendar to track events and times. The iPhone has become indispensable for Michele to remember "to do lists" and "appointments."

Michele has noticed problems with her speech since the injury (4/1/2006). She can have problem finding the correct "words to use" while talking. If she stops speaking before finishing a verbal response, she can have problems remembering where she "left off" or where "to begin." Michele enjoyed singing prior to the injury (4/1/2006). Since the injury, Michele has problems controlling her auditory perception of her vocal pitch while singing. She feels her hearing loss is the cause of her poor perception of her own vocal pitch while singing.

Michele has complaints of vertigo and disequilibrium. She has daily problems with unsteadiness and clumsiness, and quick head movements cause an acute feeling of disequilibrium and vertigo. She has felt a definite increase in a clumsy feeling since the injury. She has had disequilibrium with a sprained ankle injury on several occasions.

Michele has continuous complaints of tinnitus described as a constant ringing and an ocean, static-like. Tinnitus is always present. The tinnitus fluctuates in intensity and loudness. The tinnitus is loudest in quiet environments (i.e., night) and less bothersome (less noticeable) during the day. She listens to music to decrease and mask the background static. She had no complaints of sleep disturbance.

Michele has had headaches one (1) to two (2) per week located on the sides of the head (temples). The headaches are a continuous dull pain that can last a few hours. She usually treats headaches with OTC Advil with quick relief. The headaches were more severe if she felt aggravated or had poor sleep. Prior to the injury (4/1/2006), Michele seldom complained of headache.

Since her injury (4/01/2006), Michele has not been able to smell, and her taste has been altered. Cooking was one of her personal "passions", but now she cannot smell the foods and the taste is poor. She has experienced bad (foul) smells at times that are not present. The loss of smell results in obvious safety problems (i.e., smelling natural gas, smoke). She cannot determine whether foods are "spoiled." She has to rely on asking other family members or visual inspection or inspection of dates on container. More personally, the loss of smell and altered taste has resulted in Michele's loss of confidence in cooking. Prior to the accident, she had a passion for cooking and was a gourmet-type cook at home. She was well known by friends as an excellent Italian and Portuguese chef. Prior to the injury, Michele frequently enjoyed cooking these special meals for family and friends. The loss of smell and disturbance of taste have obviously resulted in a significant disruption of her cooking skills. She continues to cook but has to use recipes and depend on others (i.e., husband) to taste her cooking for flavor. She also must rely on family members "to watch" and "be sure" she does not burn foods when cooking. The loss of smell and alteration of taste and problems with cooking have been very aggravating to Michele's personal lifestyle.

Since the injury (4/1/2006), Michele had an episode of loss of consciousness (syncopal episode??, 4/26/2007) while she was at the Hard Rock Café (Los Angeles, CA). She was taken for immediate evaluation at Cedars-Sinai Medical Center (Los Angeles, CA). Her blood sugar was measured to be 70 mg/dl, and no definite cause of the syncopal episode was determined. She has not had additional syncopal episodes.

Michele has a complete memory loss (loss of time) for approximately two (2) days prior to the injury, no memory involving the injury on 4/1/2006, and very poor memory of events for a couple of weeks following the injury. She has noticed that she requires more sleep (at least 6 to 8 hours), or she will feel tired throughout the next day. If she does not get enough sleep, then she gets easily tired and at times emotional. She has had increased emotional irritability with family members and friends since the injury.

Michele has stopped riding her bicycle. The syncopal episode, disequilibrium, and head injury give Michele a fear of falling. She has not ridden her bicycle since the injury because of fear of an accidental fall and possible further head injury. Previously, she was an avid bicyclist.

There was no history of occupational noise exposure, recreational vehicle use or other loud noise exposure. No history of previous head injury, ear injury or severe infections. There was no previous history of hearing loss, tinnitus, vertigo or disequilibrium. There was no previous loss or alteration of smell or taste. There was no family history of hearing loss, tinnitus, or vertigo.

In sum, my inability to smell, hearing loss, balance issues, and memory shortcomings were quantified to prove that I was not 100%. However, what was true then, and especially now, is that in spite of these deficits, I was compensating for them adeptly with strengths in other areas. My physical and metaphorical backbone was intact, and it was finding new ways to connect to my nerves and limbs.

As I mentioned earlier, my sense of smell was gone, but I realized that I could taste and then recall what those things once smelled like. I could overbake a corn muffin for 35 min instead of the typical 25 because I couldn't smell it burning, and it would turn out dry and burned, instead of moist and toasty. Therefore, to solve the problem, I purchased kitchen timers that I could clip to my belt. Because I continued to cook with my new set of coping tools, dinner guests still walk in and say, "Ooh, it smells so good!" For the first 5 or 6 years since my injury, I would always correct them: "You know I can't smell!" However, now I've learned to be joyful that I can still cook so well and take pleasure in others enjoying the smells I create. I can now genuinely say, "Great!" or "Fantastic!" or "Glad to hear that!" and not mention my loss of smell at all.

My memory problems were harder at first because I was just frustrated that I couldn't come up with someone's name in 5 seconds and it instead took a minute or two. However, I finally came to accept it through a study habit I had always done but had always been embarrassed by my copious note-taking. I realized that this had always been my way to learn and succeed academically. I often got teased for taking notes in such detail because I would never be able to memorize it all. As a former cognitive psychology major, it was the encoding process of hearing/seeing and then writing it down during lectures that made me absorb the material best. Now armed with this insight after my injury, it's gone on to be a lesson I teach over and over to my students: "Find out how you learn best, some by reading, some by listening, some by writing, and some by doing, and use those learning skills as much as you can to succeed in learning."

While falls are responsible for 47% of all traumatic brain injuries, traffic accidents account for approximately 14%, according to the CDC (2013). In my circumstance, "the pedestrian versus vehicle accident" as it's referred to, there's only one likely outcome: the vehicle wins every time! My injuries, had I been thrown against the fence another way, could have been even more catastrophic. The fact that I was able to endure neurocognitive testing and pursue a lawsuit as a survivor at all was a miraculous thing.

Most TBI survivors face exorbitant medical costs: emergency services, MedeVac planes, brain surgery, additional procedures, and long recovery periods in and out of the hospital. These bills add up and begin to arrive not long after the dust settles from the traumatic event itself.

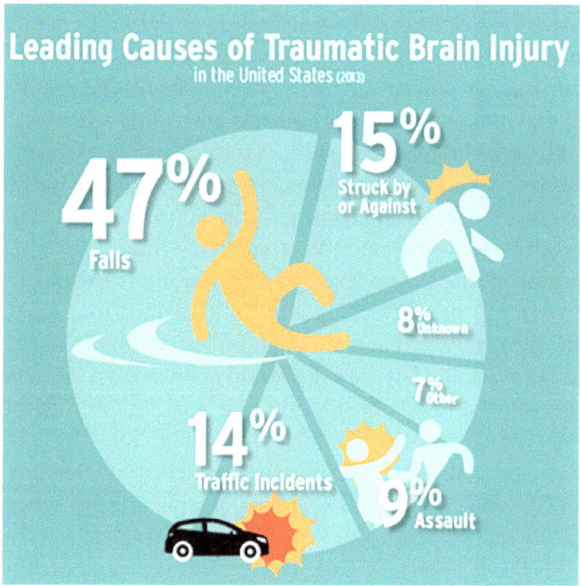

www.brainline.org*

As doctors working for both governmental and academic institutions, Carlos and I had excellent medical insurance. We were also fortunate to receive advice and resources from our friends and colleagues within the medical field when the accident occurred. The most important aspect for us was being able to reach out to colleagues and feel a sense of comfort when making decisions about which facilities and which specialists to use. This underscores the importance of having a primary provider that you know and have confidence in. They can provide this type of feedback and guidance. TBIs are unpredictable by nature, and for most people, they come as a sudden shock that they were unprepared personally or financially to care for. CNN reported that 40% of Americans cannot cover $400 for an unexpected emergency expense. * With the US healthcare system so disparate among our citizens, it is easy to see how these bills can be financially devastating to a person and their family.

For those who do not have stellar health insurance or financial resources to cover the $150,000 average cost of a brain injury in the first year*, there are a few avenues to seek relief:

- Health and accident insurance, automobile insurance
- Worker's compensation if the accident occurred while on the job
- Short- and long-term disability from your employer

Currently, crowdsourced funding allows families of victims to set up GoFundMe campaigns to receive donations immediately from anyone around the world to cover medical and legal expenses. There is also a niche industry dedicated to seeking justice (and payment) for victims if another party was involved in the accident. Some law firms that specialize in personal injury only get paid for their services if the victim recovers a settlement or judgment in their favor. For me, it was less about financial relief and more about identifying and correcting what was wrong, in principle, so that this wouldn't happen again. The elderly man who ran the stop sign at the intersection was suffering from dementia and was told by his physician that he should not drive, and more than anything, I wanted to make sure that he and others with similar disabilities would be off the road in the future.

Therefore, while doing the testing was illuminating (How much was I compensating? What were my primary complaints?), it seemed to catastrophize the outcome and label me as disabled at a time that I considered that I was doing *just fine, thank you.* For example, the lawyer's request to appear at trial in June 2009 with my head completely shaven to display my massive scar and skull deformity seemed a bridge too far for me. I loved my thick hair. I loved my job. I loved my life. For me, this legal process had outlived its usefulness. The elderly gentleman was now deeply in the throes of dementia and unable to drive, let alone the name who was president at the time ("Truman," he said). The young man had tragically passed away, which we learned from the lawyer who had tracked him down while he was still alive. Therefore, there was little satisfaction in engagement in a lengthy trial where my cognitive abilities past and present might be called into question and where the witnesses and parties were deceased or unfit to testify. This is not to say that there would not have been significant financial compensation if I had gone to trial. We were fortunate enough to not desperately need the money. This allowed us to make a choice I felt was better for my mental health, less stressful, and focused on how well I felt I was doing. A different decision by others with different financial challenges would be entirely defensible.

Therefore, our decision to settle the lawsuit was both emotional and practical. Truth is, at the age of 53, I knew that I had a lot of road left in me and a lot still to accomplish in my research and career. Rather than disclose my personal health records to go publicly to trial, I wanted the chance to earn my living and do good work. Therefore, we took a settlement rather than going to trial. We agreed to split the settlement equally among the lawyers, the insurance company, and us. Avoiding backward momentum was of the utmost importance to me.

I understand that this option is not possible for everyone and am grateful that I was able to make it.

Fresh Eyes

14

> *One who is injured ought not to return the injury, for on no account can it be right to do an injustice; and it is not right to return an injury, or to do evil to any man, however much we have suffered from him.*
>
> —Socrates, philosopher
>
> *The voyage of discovery is not in seeking new landscapes but in having new eyes.*
>
> —Marcel Proust, author

In the previous chapter, I described the persistent challenges of the first 3–4 years after my TBI event. As I now review that timeframe more than 10 years later, I am struck by changes I had not even noticed: things that appeared in the assessment of my injuries when I was still pursing the lawsuit that I no longer pay attention to. It isn't that I don't still have those deficits but perhaps more that I have either compensated or gotten used to them. I must admit that I see things through different, fresh eyes now.

The headaches just went away, and in fact it is only in reading the report from 2009 that I am reminded I even had them! As a psychiatrist, I wonder if the headaches were not just from my head trauma but also anxiety and frustration over my recovery not going fast enough. I'm not known for my patience! However, once I convinced myself that I had recovered, perhaps I relaxed or stopped noticing the headaches at all.

Vertigo and disequilibrium are both examples of "getting used to it" and compensation. My testing for the neuro-otology report showed that while I had some vertigo, more of my problems with balance occurred because I wasn't or wouldn't pay as much attention. There are three things that affect your balance: one is your eyes that look down or ahead to the horizon to help you compensate for changes that are occurring in your environment. The other is the neuromuscular signals that come from your feet, legs, and sometimes whole body. It's like watching a soccer player maintain their balance even when they stumble on the field. The third is the semicircular canals, three of them, in each ear. They are similar to the x, y, and z of graph paper in three dimensions. They help you as you move around to keep your head and body balanced. However, these semicircular canals on each side of your head, in the inner most part of each ear (one in each hemisphere), are close to your brain and often damaged in some way during TBI. My balance testing in this 2009 report showed that I had good balance overall for my age but that I made many more compensations than typical for someone my age. On a positive note, I attribute this to all my years in childhood and early adulthood playing soccer on very uneven and grass-gouged fields. Being an avid long-distance runner, I always look down at the road ahead, and I rarely if ever trip. However, as an animated talker and proud Italian, as I've mentioned before, I always talk and move my hands, even while I am walking. My vision is not always able to help my neuromuscular cues and my semicircular canal defects. Therefore, I often twist my ankles when walking. While I catch myself, like stepping in a grass "pothole" on the soccer field or on cobblestone sidewalks, I also always carry an ace bandage in my pocketbook and suitcase wherever I go!

These are lessons I've learned along the way to "get by", and in the advent of time, I realize that I truly view my TBI differently than I did back then. After all, we all compensate for things we lose as we age. However, that usually happens more gradually as opposed to how swiftly the TBI took those away for me: do we truly have any choice but to compensate?

The loss of smell is an example of compensation and finding enjoyment in what I can still do. It was a relief to be able to enjoy cooking even though it was aggravating to have to remind people I could not smell. I would be off shopping in some specialty store and my friend would say, "Here, smell this basil or cinnamon," and I felt compelled to correct them that I can't smell. However, over the first 8 years, I have changed my tune, and I see it differently now that I have found ways to compensate. As I mentioned earlier, I've come to embrace the high compliment for my fragrant cooking. Then, I started to notice that when I tasted something, it would "remind" me of what it smelled like. After all, the cranial nerves that contribute to smell and taste are related. So now my husband lets me be the "wine taster" at the table when we go out just to prove I can use my sense of taste to help me "smell"! It may not be quite the same as both smelling and tasting, but I can use my imagination. My taste in wine has changed somewhat, but when a friend hands me an herb to smell in their kitchen now, I say, "Ohhh, let me put it on my tongue to smell it!" It's become a running joke among friends and so much more enjoyable for everyone.

Hearing loss is a more common deficit since it is a gradual symptom associated with aging. Like many people who have experienced it, I am often reluctant to acknowledge the decline. I was once an avid singer and enjoyed live music and singalongs, but hearing loss is a subtle killer. I first noticed it when I would give large group presentations, like my grand rounds or research events where I would insist on a microphone not just for me but for the audience so I could field audience questions, so that I could hear what they asked. I learned to become more diligent in these scenarios by repeating the questions asked as well, which is not a bad habit for a public speaker! For me, although, it was more to make sure I had heard the question correctly.

This didn't *truly* get under my skin until I was lecturing to my own psychiatry residents. Even with a repeated request to speak up, I could not get them to project their questions or their comments to my own questions. This was especially true among my female residents, since that higher frequency of hearing was most damaged as a result of my head trauma. Early in their residency, I tried to give a lecture on TBI and use my own MRI images and experiences in the lecture, but still I was having trouble. Finally, approximately 8 years after my head injury, I got ReSound hearing aids that were specially programmed to deal with my areas of deficits. They are Bluetooth coupled to my iPhone and therefore instantly modulate to my surroundings. I continue to wear these hearing aids today and get them refitted and adjusted often. I still wish some of the quieter female residents would just speak up! I now rely on these hearing aids so much that I'm shocked about how long it took me to get them. Maybe it was my own stubbornness or the stigma of wearing hearing aids. That said, I truly encourage anyone who experiences hearing loss to consider this option. Technology has come a long way, and most kinds are barely perceptible to others. My hearing aids don't even show. When I take them off and on and show them to people, they are always shocked that they are there. I even convinced my mom when she turned 82 to get the ReSound hearing aids.

The tinnitus that I reported back in 2009 is a distant memory. Luckily, I don't have this anymore and I don't even recall complaining about it, although I'm sure I did. When you have that constant ringing in your ear on top of the hearing loss, it makes what others are saying to you even more difficult to comprehend. I don't know for sure that my hearing has deteriorated that much. For some people, tinnitus can fade over time, and for others, it remains. I am not sure why it stopped being a persistent issue for me, and I still have it sometimes, but I just try to ignore it. About once a month I may experience a buzzing sound when in a quiet room trying to fall asleep.

When reflecting on and writing about my deficits outlined in that report, it shows me how a TBI will alter your perspective immensely. Even now I find the process of reading about them difficult and uncomfortable, but I've chosen to accept that it's how I once was and felt. Miraculously, eyesight was among the senses not affected by my head injury. Coming to terms with yourself after such an event is a big step in the process. The passage of time is another. I'm feeling grateful that when I look in the mirror, I still see Michele and I've found innovative ways to continue being myself.

Wings

15

I cannot change the direction of the wind, but I can adjust my sails to always reach my destination.

—Jimmy Dean, businessman

If you know where you are from, it will be harder for people to stop you where you are going.

—Matshona Dhliwayo, author

Life runs its natural course, and things keep moving forward and changing. If you are standing still, it is truly like going backward. Think about this for a minute: does it make sense? Imagine swimming in a river against a current. Anytime you stop paddling, you lose ground. So as someone who is in constant motion, this is something that always happens to me. As I have already explained, I was a squirmy kid, and someone "who just couldn't sit still." In first grade, in Catholic school, Sister Vincent Fiera was never bothered by this. Instead, she just kept putting new challenges in front of me, giving me new books to read. I read over 50 extra books besides those assigned in class. In second grade, the "lay" class teacher, Mrs. Berry, told my parents during a parent-teacher conference that while I was a good student, she thought I should stop raising my hand so other kids would have an opportunity to answer. While it may have been a compliment that she thought I knew all the answers, it absolutely stifled my can't-sit-still attitude. I never raised my hand because I wanted to be show-off; I was just that gung ho about learning that I couldn't share my answer. Later that year, I had entered the science fair by building an electromagnet, and so did another boy in my grade. I won first place because I was better able to explain how it worked. Ironically, they awarded me first place but did not give me the first-place prize, a chemistry set, since they didn't think that it was "appropriate" for a *girl*! Instead, I got the third-place prize, a statue of the Virgin Mary. I still have that statue to this day, but I must admit there is a little ding in her halo (literally and figuratively). It's no wonder that I first decided to pursue a chemistry major at Brown University. I was probably still thinking about that chemistry set I never got!

Even though it wasn't always in my favor, I have always pushed the envelope and bucked the tide. Ten years after my head injury in 2015, Carlos, my partner in all of life for 40 years, and I made the decision to move our academic careers forward and take on a new challenge. He became the dean of a medical school (he was formerly the chair of psychiatry), and I was the head of a new genetics institute, the Institute for Genomic Health, which I was very excited about. Rather than just studying genes that are linked to specific illnesses, it was an initiative that focused on how genes affect your well-being too. I like to say, "genes don't just make you sick, they keep you healthy."

Even though I had moved on in so many ways, the most important question remained unanswered: *why?* Why had I recovered, and as a doctor, what could I learn to help others recover better? Perhaps this is why I chose to align myself with other psychiatric experts in traumatic brain injury from the years 2012 to 2015. I was part of four yearly seminars at the American Psychiatric Association (APA) that discussed TBI in civilians, athletes, and soldiers. For my part in these 3-h seminars, I talked about ssTBI (single severe TBI), which is typically seen in the civilian—child, adult, or elderly adult—and often caused by a fall or a motor vehicle accident. I used my own MRIs and photos, some of which I've included in this book, to both humanize and personalize the experience. It felt good to share my recovery and show what was possible even after such a devastating injury. It was vital to send the message not to give up! However, I still wanted to do more. After all, my initial prognosis had been guarded and predicted significant disability. In attempting to give us reasonable expectations, we were told that I might speak at a child's level, maybe dress myself, and follow simple commands. However, within 4 weeks of my injury, postcranioplasty (the repair of my skull), I was talking and a week after that typing email responses on my laptop computer. If something like this *had* to happen to someone, perhaps it wasn't so terrible that it had happened to me. If I could use my position as a lecturer and mentor to then teach about TBI from the patient's perspective in the future, maybe that's how things were meant to be.

At the time, the move to State University of New York Downstate (SUNY Downstate) in July 2015 revealed something new. When I got to SUNY Downstate, I was not immediately recognized as someone who had survived a brain injury. At USC, my colleagues were shocked to see that I was alive and talking. It was like walking around with a tattoo on my forehead. It wasn't that I was damaged goods, but I could feel that there was an underlying concern among colleagues about my cognitive functioning. It was particularly embarrassing when one of the faculty members at USC wanted to know if the rough draft of a manuscript I had sent had grammatical issues because of my past TBI.

With this in mind, I think that the advantage of moving to Brooklyn after being in California for so long (10 years) was that 90% of the psychiatrists I met would not know about my head injury. Either they were not part of my inner circle or were not active in organizations such as the AAP, AADPRT, or APA, where they might have run across me or seen one of my previous TBI talks. Thus, they just judged me as the psychiatrist I was, and not as the brain-injured wife of the chair of psychiatry at USC. So even though I was somewhat coming back "home" to New York, it was also a bit of a fresh start.

Having grown up on Long Island, I was familiar with the expressways and bridges of New York. However, Brooklyn is a different animal than the rest of the island. It has its own sense of place and feel, as many New Yorkers can attest to how insular and unique parts of the city and its boroughs can be. I was coming home to the fast-paced, fast-talking culture that I was so comfortable with. Out in California I had to deliberately slow myself down, whereas I can talk just as fast as I want here in New York, and no one bats an eye or misses a beat! I was also able to reconnect to some of my colleagues, such as psychiatrist Shari Luskin, epidemiologist Evelyn Bromet, and psychiatric geneticist Dolores Malaspina. While I left a lot back in California, there were opportunities living in New York to look forward to.

At Downstate, I continued to promote research and was made vice chair for research and research training for residents and faculty in the psychiatry department. We also converted a newly renovated but vacant inpatient space into an outpatient research center with ten rooms to conduct studies. In addition to these developments, I continued to give grand rounds, teach residents, and take on a medical student "intern" for each summer. I gave a lecture on TBI at Downstate, but it wasn't until January of 2017, 18 months after arriving at SUNY Downstate, that I gave a grand round lecture about TBI. Instead of collaborating with two other experts, I did the lecture on my own, not revealing to the audience ahead of time about my TBI. I only revealed that the talk was a "personal narrative."

The lecture hall was packed. As the dean, Carlos introduced me, and I began with the first slide: this is an MRI of a normal brain. *Click*. This is a brain with a single severe traumatic brain injury. *Click*. This was *my* brain. It was me. To some in the audience, residents and colleagues who had known me since I came to Downstate, this was the first time hearing my story, and it came as a real shock. They were in the medical field, and they could see just how catastrophic the damage was. As I showed another slide, a photo of me after waking up from coma, I could sense the room collectively gasp. Although I was pictured smiling in the hospital bed, the left side of my head was missing, a huge chunk of negative space. It is important to note that both my mom and son Eric came and sat in the front row with Carlos. It was a pivotal moment. Eric filmed the whole lecture and question and answer session on his iPhone. I asked mom a few questions from the podium about my injury and recovery, but she was too teary-eyed and uncharacteristically tongue-tied by the experience to say much. During the Q&A, Carlos helped answer questions about the accident, especially those details that I could not remember. It is common for a grand round lecture to clear out after the main lecture concludes, but nearly everyone in the audience stayed in their seats to hear more. It was this presentation that allowed me to fully appreciate how sharing my story could help others, whether they are patients, colleagues, family, or friends.

One resident commented, "Very touching report…truly amazing recovery and I never would have suspected. I'm curious when you were in the hospital you were [having] a lot of communication with your husband and your family and you could not express yourself. I'm curious if there was anyone at the hospital, staff member or somebody who does not know you who was good at connecting with you? Reassuring you, giving you a sense that you could communicate?" My answer was yes and no—that Carlos was the one who helped communicate with and for me, although some of the therapists did their best and helped me do more during physical therapy. Another person said, "Michele, thank you so much for taking us on your personal journey. It is a journey through resilience. This room was standing room only and I've never seen that. So that is a testament." One resident wondered, "This is a very frightening situation. What truly kept you going?" To which I answered, "I'm just a very persistent person. Why do you think I study OCD? Study what you know!" There was a burst of laughter in the room, and I then discussed the Connor-Davidson Resilience Scale and the 25 questions associated with it. I concluded by saying, "However, I think what's more important is to say it varies with the individual and that is why understanding more about what [the patient was] like before becomes valuable. I had to push my therapists to listen to my family. You know, they know me! It is very important and Carlos did get accused of being too involved, but it truly made a difference."

The difficulty in sharing something as personal as a brain injury is that you must contend with the magnitude of your own survival. There are gaps created by trauma, be it a medically induced coma or memory loss. To know what happened has been such a critical part of my story that took many years, and the course of writing this book, to fill in. I will never be 100% certain of what happened, but I do know that I have recovered. As I said in the lecture, Carlos still corrects me when I misspeak or use the wrong word, but I am 95% recovered, and that's a feat in and of itself.

Therefore, after years keeping my head down and pushing onward, now the cat was out of the bag, and I could see the value and impact of sharing my TBI story. One of the final questions, "Everything you've gone through sounds like a medical miracle. I wondered if you have become a case study yourself?" I answered, "I'm working on it!"

Lungs

16

*Breathe deeply, until sweet air extinguishes the burn of fear in
your lungs and every breath is a beautiful refusal to become
anything less than infinite.*

—D. Antoinette Foy

The most difficult decision is to act, the rest is merely tenacity.

—Amelia Earhart, pilot

Not everyone has the unique opportunity to reflect on their own resilience. It seems
to me, these many years out from the injury, that my compensatory skills and general
stubbornness have served me well through my TBI. Although I've never personally
described myself as "tenacious," one person used that word in reaction to
my grand rounds lecture at SUNY Downstate, and it seems to be true. Tenacity is all
about hanging in there especially when the chips are down. While I study OCD,
which means persistence is on a whole other level for me, it seems that these principles
are universal. If I could have something to add to the research and awareness
surrounding TBI, it would make the most sense to use what I've learned in the process
for the good of others. It's the reason I then gave a talk at Stony Brook University
that focused even more on my own TBI.

First off, it's important to acknowledge that merely "surviving" was never going
to satisfy me. Breathing is vital and essential, but my definition of survival included
cognition and the ability to think. Carlos and I already agreed that quality of life
meant having a working brain, and that had things gone differently, I might not be
here writing this book. Therefore, I am fortunate to have beaten the odds at the outset
of my injury. Others who suffer a brain injury may not be able to do this. They
may be in coma for a longer amount of time than I was, or the swelling on the brain
might affect different areas and corresponding abilities. However, that doesn't mean
they couldn't improve or make progress, however small or incremental. Life teaches

© The Author(s), under exclusive license to Springer Nature Switzerland AG 2023   93
M. T. Pato, *Nerve*, https://doi.org/10.1007/978-3-031-33433-7_16

us that the road is often long and bumpy. Patients with TBI should be considered as the individuals they were beforehand, setting goals and expectations based upon what was important or significant about them before the accident. We know that aphasias prevent patients from properly communicating but that the intent and thought behind the communication is still with the person, even though they are not able to express themselves. Therefore, it is important to never underestimate what a patient (in coma or conscious) may or may not understand about the world around them. Playing music they loved, reading out loud, holding their hand, and surrounding them with familiar things go a long way. As I mentioned earlier, these were some of the things my family did for me when I was in and out of the hospital, and it was a game changer.

What I find interesting (and disappointing) about researching TBI and trying to write about it is that not much is known or "out there" about long-term outcomes. Neurosurgeons do not follow their patients 5, 10, or 20 years after the injury. An article titled "Aging After Brain Injury: BrainLine Talks with Dr. Steven Flanagan" discusses the potential of developing further cognitive issues such as seizures, early-onset Parkinson's disease, and dementia.

He also acknowledges the shortcomings of the current TBI research:

> Ideally, we need to have a long-term study that looks at how brain injury affects cognition as a person gets older. For example, if we could study the cognitive skills of people with brain injury versus those without brain injury at 30 years of age and then at 60 years of age, we would probably learn a great deal. However, that kind of study is almost impossible because it is difficult to follow people for so many years.
> That said, people with brain injury, especially those with long-term cognitive issues, should stay in touch with their doctor, preferably a physician knowledgeable about brain injury.

I'm not sure how many primary care doctors are truly knowledgeable about brain injury, and I'm saying that as a doctor myself! Whenever I go to see my primary care doctor or even a massage therapist, I have to remind him or her of my past history. This is even harder to do when you only get an average of 15 min to visit with your doctor. Therefore, with this being our current healthcare system, we have to advocate for ourselves. In many countries with universal healthcare, this is not the case. Instead of "sick care" (meaning only going to the doctor when you are ill), they promote regular annual checkups and prevention.

For example, Dr. Flanagan suggests following up one or two times a year with their doctor about their past TBI. However, it is very revealing that in the comments section of the BrainLine article, there are multiple comments about how people or their loved ones did not get or have access to long-term follow-up treatment. * It seems by the nature of the dialog that many TBI survivors came to the site looking for answers related to living with TBI and ended up sharing their personal stories in pursuit of further support. Clearly, there is much more to be learned and done to help those who continue to live with their TBIs.

In fact I had to suggest, no, insist on, getting an MRI scan of my brain, after 12 years, taken so I could see how my brain might have changed or declined in the years since. Aside from having to fight for the MRI, it was also a difficult personal decision to get a brain scan. What would we find? How much had changed or gotten worse? After living life with my TBI for this long, did I need more hard evidence of my injury?

The answer, as you may have guessed by now, was *yes*, I needed to know. The decision was not made lightly, and I truly struggled over the course of several weeks before coming to terms with it. The bottom line was this: if something was new or surprising, it was possible that I could still do something about it. They make preventative drugs like Aricept to delay or slow dementia in elderly patients, and if there was a way for me to improve or stave off big changes, I would. Therefore, in 2018, I had another MRI done. Then, I sent a DVD of my MRIs (April 26, 2006, and April 26, 2018) to a neuroradiologist colleague and friend to read and interpret them. In her professional opinion, which I also asked her to then explain in lay terms, this is what she had to say:

***

I did get a chance to look at the new DVD and compare it with the old images. There has been interval involution of previously seen large hemorrhagic contusive injuries involving the medial anterior margins of the bilateral frontal lobes as well as the lateral anterior margin of the left temporal lobe. There are focal areas of cystic encephalomalacia involving the bilateral frontal lobes, more extensive on the left. There is prominent gliosis involving the left temporal lobe with corresponding peripheral hemosiderin staining.

There are additional punctate white matter foci within the periventricular and subcortical white matter, without corresponding hemosiderin staining. These may be related to nonhemorrhagic shear injuries or chronic small vessel ischemic disease.

In lay terms, this means the large areas of blood in the brain have shrunk. Fluid collections have replaced the portions of the brain that were injured and died as a result of the injury. Scarring is also seen along the margins of the injured brain matter. Some broken down blood products remain at the area of prior injury. [Areas of the brain that were injured include those that control cognitive function, language, memory, comprehension, sensory input, and emotion.]

Some changes seen deeper in the brain matter could have resulted from the original shearing injury that occurred as the brain shifted and rotated in the skull. These findings could also have resulted from changes to the small vessels in the brain that can develop with aging.

I have to say that it is truly miraculous that Michele is so highly functioning. Writing a book after all this...amazing! Does she have some issues with memory? The extent of injury to the bilateral frontal lobes would be concerning for personality changes as well as difficulties with memory. Is she treated for seizures? Gliosis along the left temporal lobe would be a potential seizure focus.

***

The neuroradiologist's questions about memory and personality issues remind me of how lucky I am that I only struggle to remember names! Although I wouldn't outright dismiss her specific concerns, it further demonstrates how much my brain has found a way around the existing damage. Recent studies on the brain's plasticity show that you can continue to learn and grow even as you age. The brain works in mysterious ways!

My TBI journey started when I was 50 years old, arguably at the peak of my career, and has led me to contemplate the ways in which I continue to live and age with my TBI. It's one thing to overcome the initial injury, but it's another to truly live with it. In addition, I do. Like drawing breath, it becomes an automatic function. However, there are reminders everywhere of what I used to be able to do without a second thought that I now do with caution or simply avoid. Although I would never truly admit I avoid them, that would be a sign of giving into my limitations, but I do find some interesting workarounds.

I can't walk into the street against a light and definitely no jaywalking! This may not sound like much, but it's a rarity in NYC and its five boroughs for pedestrians to obey traffic signals. As a driver, it makes me "crazy" to have to honk or drive around people who are standing in the street and not on the sidewalk waiting to cross. I swear pedestrians must think you can stop on a dime since they often cross the street wherever they please! I can reflect on the irony that I was standing on the sidewalk, waiting for a traffic signal when I was struck by the car. When other pedestrians are impatiently waiting with me for the signal to give us permission to cross, I say, "Is it worth getting hit by a car?" Sometimes it calms them down, especially if I mention I'm a TBI survivor, but sometimes they become annoyed! When I'm grabbing a taxi, it's hard not to rush in as everyone does, but I have to be careful not to bump my head, as I have a few times!

As I've mentioned earlier, I avoid activities and sports where I could possibly reinjure my brain. Skiing again remains a great hope of mine; however, I'm not sure that Carlos will allow it. (Sometimes our loved ones help remind us of our limitations too.) I can't take amusement park rides either, although this hasn't been a big problem for me. Growing up, my sister and mom got carsick, so I would be the one to go on all the amusement rides with dad or other family. Sometimes my sister would go if she was feeling brave. Then, with my two boys, now 33 and 35, it was never a question! Of course, we would go on all the rides. I already miss the idea that I won't be able to do the rollercoasters with my granddaughter, or some of the jolting haunted house rides, but then I think okay, I'll stick to the boat rides and railroads driving through imagined towns. If worse comes to worse, I'll hold everyone's bags and coats and take the pictures as they scream with joy and fright as they zoom by me.

Apart from the everyday concerns, there's a nagging question of whether something I am experiencing is normal aging or a result of my injury. It may mean I need to get my hearing aids adjusted more often or be vigilant with checking in with myself and how I'm doing.

Recently, I've been experiencing some annoying neck pain and finger numbness in my right and sometimes left hand, which has led me to question the source. Therefore, after 8 months of it getting worse, I got an MRI of my neck done, wondering if was I experiencing neck issues because of my TBI? Nope, it was normal. In the end, it turned out to be carpal tunnel syndrome in both wrists, which is something that just "runs" in my family. My mom has it and has gotten successful treatment and now I'm doing the same.

Like many women, I consulted with my OB/GYN about hormone therapy before I hit menopause but after my TBI. There was evidence at the time that taking estrogen-progesterone would stave off dementia and many of the symptoms associated with menopause. However, with some new research in the past 2–3 years, we discovered that the risk of cancer increases, and the cognitive benefits are slim. It made sense to go off of them after 13 years. Once the decision was made, I began to experience menopause rapidly and wonder if some of these physical issues, like hot flashes, have something to do with the choice to stop? Most likely, but it will always be a thought, is this because of my TBI injury? This is what I mean when I say I didn't overcome the TBI exactly, but rather *I live* with it. Consciously and subconsciously, it is a part of your life forever.

There are plenty of ways in which the body is predictable. Every breath we draw is automatically regulated by the autonomic nervous system (ANS), and it takes real mental focus to attempt to change it. I can't do anything about what happened to my brain so many years ago, but I can be proactive about my health and adapt as I get older. My TBI is a fact of life, and my inherent resilience is the reason I can cope with the challenge and continue to live in a way that I choose.

Gut

17

I can be changed by what happens to me. However, I refuse to be reduced by it.

—Maya Angelou, poet

Never ignore a gut feeling, but never believe it is enough.

—Robert Heller, management guru

Writing this account of my injury and the years since has given me profound purpose. Just as I once asked the question, "Why did this happen to me?", I continue to ponder how I can make a real difference to other TBI patients and their families. It is staggering and unsettling how much we still do not know about these injuries and their long-term outcomes. As I mentioned earlier, scientists cannot study a single severe traumatic brain injury the same way you can other diseases and illnesses. There is no way to replicate a head injury; each is totally unpredictable and unique. There's also no precedent for the manner in which I was able to be treated; the swelling was so extreme and the response so fast (within 30 min) that I may be the outlier in an otherwise bleak graph. I don't take this for granted. However, my gut tells me that what I experienced could benefit other patients in the future.

When people are faced with an extreme illness or injury, time stands still. Your life stops, your friends' and family's lives stop, and all hands are on deck to make sure you survive. That's where all the focus is. However, one day, hopefully, you will acclimate to real life again. That may mean that you do some of what you used to with physical or medical aids or that you relearn what your daily routines or skills are. Whatever your new reality is, it's undeniable that the process of healing from a brain injury is ongoing.

As much as I may have recovered and thrived, my TBI never leaves me. It hovers over me, whether I am conscious of it or not. Recently, I was working on writing and submitting an important grant with our team of colleagues, and things were coming

M. T. Pato, *Nerve*, https://doi.org/10.1007/978-3-031-33433-7_17

down to the 11th hour. We had differences of opinion with one researcher who was holding out for certain conditions, and it was taking 30 min of an hour-long conference call. I had been good and kept quiet for so long, until one moment when I just blurted out, "Shut up! You can have what you want!" Carlos was upset with me for saying it, and I do wonder in hindsight if that was some sort of frontal lobe disinhibition creeping in from my TBI. There's no way for me to know for sure, but that seed of doubt never completely goes away.

This raises an especially important issue when we consider how brain injuries are managed throughout the rest of a person's life. They should be prioritized in the same way as chronic diseases such as diabetes, ADHD, dementia, or autoimmune conditions such as Crohn's, lupus, or multiple sclerosis. TBI history should always be at the top of the patient's chart and be factored into how other diseases, illnesses, or health issues are treated. One common side effect of TBI is an alteration of the personality and/or regulation of emotions. This makes mental health a major area of concern, and more research should be done to better understand the relationship between head injuries and psychology. One excellent resource for articles can be found at *https://www.lapublishing.com/blog/*. Most of the pieces are short, easy to read, and written by people who continue to cope with TBI. In addition, each piece offers other resources and publications to turn to for more information if you are interested.

I must recommend further reading the compelling account of author Kara L. Swanson's closed head injury in a 1996 car accident, which while diagnosed as mild, rather than severe like mine, was never symptomatically mild since she suffered from severe balance issues, short-term memory issues, career loss, and mood fluctuations. She details her immediate physical and mental health recovery in *I'll Carry the Fork!* and has subsequently published a 20th anniversary update. Her blog, which continues to be a source of support for the TBI community, can be found at karaswanson.wordpress.com. Another TBI survivor, David A. Grant, has written *Metamorphosis: Surviving Brain Injury* and continues to write at *http://surviving-brain-injury.blogspot.com/ about his TBI and other relevant topics today.*

I'm not the only one with TBI to talk about change and improvement continuing for years and not reaching an endpoint when you leave the hospital (David A. Grant 2015-Metamorphosis, Surviving Brain Injury—Chap. 15—Permanently Disabled?). Perhaps improvement seems a little too optimistic for some. After all certain injuries like my loss of smell haven't truly improved at all, yet what time has done has allowed me to find ways to adapt with my other senses. So now even though I can't smell, I can taste, and finally after 15 years I can smile when people walk into my kitchen and tell me it smells great. I am happy I can cook things that smell good even though I can't smell it. My friends have adapted too. Walking through the herb garden of my friend just 2 weeks ago, she leans down and grabs some exotic mint and says "Smell this." I immediately say is it okay to taste, and she says "Oh yeah sure" (she keeps an organic garden so I was pretty sure there were not pesticides). And I taste and say "Wow, great, what do you put it in!"

So perhaps this is not different from how one adapts with age and experience, but having survived TBI, I am extra aware and so I have gained appreciation for what I still have and how to continue to use it in new ways. As Grant notes, following his cognitive psych testing which was less than optimistic: (pg. 203) "What it did not reveal, however was that I was on a road and not at a final resting point……please be mindful that a single snapshot does not take into consideration what the future will hold. Neural plasticity is a wonderful, amazing and little understood part of the healing process as the brain finds new ways to do what used to be familiar."

Even though there are some great accounts of TBI out there now, I remain unconvinced that we have done enough for the TBI community. Further research needs to be done, and consideration must be made for each individual patient through personalized medicine.

Case in point, the professional textbook for traumatic brain injury, written by Jonathan M. Silver and others, is extensive at 807 pages but only has 1 chapter dedicated to "Activities, Participation, and Community Integration," wherein some case examples and their long-term outcomes are discussed and social integration encouraged. Therapies, treatment, and emotions are discussed in the other chapters, as well as special populations, but it is notable that there is not much out there discussing TBIs several years out from the injury. This falls miles short of where we should be. I believe that living a life with TBI should never truly reach a plateau but should always be about taking the next step. Yes, we all age, but special attention should be given to the person with TBI. They are all different (no two are exactly alike), but it is important to find common ground and empathy toward those who are affected.

Empathy is about understanding what others feel without any judgment, approval, or criticism. I discovered that empathy comes with practice. Just recently, I was trying to study empathy in the context of medicine, not just to make myself a better doctor but to help those who are suffering with anxiety and stress. One of my fellow residents and a friend/colleague who I trained with back in 1984–1986, Helen Riess, MD, has written a book called *The Empathy Effect*. She has also developed a face-to-face (F2F) and online program at Massachusetts General Hospital (MGH) on empathy and a Consortium for Research on Emotional Intelligence and has taught to organizations around the world. Once again, I have become a student of something new and a teacher for others. In her book, she describes what empathy is and how you can learn and improve your use of it.

The seven letters of EMPATHY tell you what you need to do to develop empathy with another person: E is for eye contact with the other person and M is for observing how they move their facial muscles, especially around the mouth and eyes. This tells you so much about what they are feeling. P is for posture—how do they hold themselves, how do they bend their neck, or how are they sitting. A is for affect—what emotion are you feeling from them—they may say they are happy with the smile in their mouth, but their eyes may show sadness instead, so what is the conflict they are feeling. T is for tone—the way their voice sounds can often tell you more than the words that come out of their mouth. The H is for hearing what the person says, and in fact their choice of words or what they choose not to say is something that can tell you a lot about the unspoken words of empathy. The final letter Y is for you and your reaction. This means regulating how you respond to someone to show you understand their feelings and not judge them with your own. Perhaps one of the key things about empathy is applying it to oneself. Self-empathy is not about being selfish but allowing the same nonjudgmental understanding that you give to another person to yourself, your reactions, and your actions. Forgiving shortcomings is one way that I have learned to be kinder to myself over the years following my TBI.

In any kind of medicine, it is truly important to listen and truly hear what the patient is saying. With every patient, there is a chief *complaint*, or the reason they are seeing you ("Doc, I have a face rash!"), and an underlying chief *concern* ("I can't go to work looking like this!"), which could be the greater issue that needs to be addressed to make the person feel better. Hearing not only the chief complaint but also finding the chief concern is a way to utilize empathy. In my own recovery, one of my chief *complaints* was that I couldn't smell and how would I know when something was burning or when fruit had turned rotten? Although I had lost my sense of smell and knew the olfactory neurons would probably not grow back, my chief *concern* was could I still cook and enjoy those activities with others, which was such a big part of my life? My doctors understood this was my concern, perhaps enough to let me out on furlough just around day 22 or 24, although it never would have happened without the cajoling of my husband, to cook my first dinner for my family since my injury. What about the other components of EMPATHY? What about the nonverbal cues, like what I saw with my eyes when I finally opened them, and how I smiled with the muscles of my face, or how I held my head when sitting with those who visited (my *posture*), or how I laughed (my *affect*) and how that laugh or that singing voice sounded (my *tone*), and finally in hearing what others were saying to me, how I responded? These are the pieces of EMPATHY that I brought to my recovery and used to communicate and regain my sense of belonging. Empathy is a part of caring for ourselves and caring for others, be they family, friends, or patients. It is a vital part of being human and belonging in a social world.

I have had to challenge myself to appreciate and understand other survivors who have gone through this journey, which will be similar and different at the same time. While I have reached a place of acceptance with my own injury and recovery, it's hard to know exactly how others in my family feel about it. I was too busy going through it, so I did not share their countless hours of worry and caretaking. Interestingly, it has been difficult to jog some of their specific memories of the accident, even though they definitely remember more than I did of that day! For my mother, the process of reliving the event seems to be too painful for her to bear. During the one lecture that she attended when I shared my story with residents and faculty, it rendered her speechless, which is nearly impossible! When I asked her about why she didn't have anything to add when prompted, she reminded me that she had never seen some of the extreme images of my brain and head. She claimed it was because I had never shown them to her in the past, and I asked her if that upset her. She replied, "You know when we were all in the hospital Daddy [my father] and Michael would go into the room and just come out crying." This must have been while I was still in coma and everyone was camped out in waiting room. She continued, "Eric would go in and out smiling and say it's Mom, you know she is going to fight this and survive." His gut feeling knew, whatever it was, I would face it and come out all right on the other side. That optimism seems extraordinary given the bleakness of the moment, but I have no doubt some of that positive attitude influenced my recovery.

While both sons grew up with two doctors at the dinner table, they organized their own learning in different ways. For Michael, it was the science and analysis of data and computer technology that made him creative. For Eric, it was art, which started with the medium of pencil and paper and then paint and canvas, and now it's computer/digital. Both find creative and uplifting ways to interpret data. Perhaps Eric could conjure me up with his mind's eye and see what I would be. Even while seeing me, even in my damaged state, could make him smile, rather than cry, more easily. Eric was never just seeing what was in front of his eyes but using his creativity and imagination and memories from the past to "see" what I would be like in the future.

On the other hand, Carlos may take a view that because I have remained largely the same Michele in his eyes, there is no reason to dwell on what happened. However, for me, writing this account has been quite therapeutic. For one, reconstructing the timeline and order of events surrounding the accident took some enormous effort and digging through reports, medical records, and notes. I must thank Ana Pato Morley and her husband Chris for journaling, writing, and blogging about it all in such detail. Without that contemporaneous account of my progress, I wouldn't have been able to remember (or in some cases, discover!) much about those early days.

You'll notice that I have included a few pictures about my progress during recovery. You can see how much my brain shifted and how the swelling went into my ventricles. In addition, you can see how dented my head looked and how big my scar was and (still) is. However, to be honest there are few pictures of the first 18 months. I truly had to hunt for many of the ones I've included here. As I think back on this, I suspect that those like me who have recovered took few pictures along the way. At the time, it seems horrible to remember how "damaged" we look and feel. Maybe this is why my mother had so much trouble speaking at my grand rounds presentation when she finally saw some of these pictures. Now, as I reflect back on the years, I am so glad I have those pictures because when I have doubt and worry that I am not continuing to recover, they remind me of how far I have come. As they say, one picture is worth a thousand words!

The process of putting it all together in book form has necessarily been a long one. However, in the time it has taken to do so, I have reached profound acceptance, perspective, and even gratitude for my TBI. It is especially encouraging that despite earlier beliefs that the brain is in a constant state of decline after reaching maturity, it is not a fixed entity. It changes over time and can adapt to a multitude of challenges, even one as severe as brain injury. As I have discussed the ways my brain has found creative workarounds for its deficits and how to use resilience and empathy to overcome hurdles, I have also discovered that the autonomic nervous system (ANS) can also be trained in some ways.

As it happens, a medical student who is running a study on the ANS using heart rate variability and respiratory rate variability has recently taken me on as a subject. It will be fascinating to learn how my own system, after all I've been through, performs. We all have variations in our heart rate (heart rate variability, HRV), which is the space between each heartbeat. Consider this example: two people run up a steep hill. One perhaps exercises regularly and the other does not. At the top of the hill, one person is out of breath and takes a long time to return to a normal resting heart rate. The other's heart rate bounces back from the high rate to resting quicker. This is heart rate variability, and although it is a part of the ANS, which operates automatically, you can learn how to better control it. Breathing (respiratory rate variability, RRV) is another factor that can be changed with practice. For instance, deep breathing from the diaphragm is one way we can alter our natural rhythms of our heart and respiration. By changing our breathing, we can learn to change the heart's variability and thereby help calm ourselves down from a panicked or anxious state.

Meditation is another way to manage stress. While I was in college studying, I used to take "power" naps where I would put myself in a trance, or immediate REM state, to get the most out of those 15–20 min before resuming my coursework. I also used this meditation technique while giving birth to both of my sons, unmedicated. Breathing and mental exercises can slow and regulate the "automatic" heartbeat and breathing, which gives us a way to manage stress or get through physical or emotional pain.

Whether you are fighting a battle with anxiety or struggling to regain a life after TBI, there is hope out there. The body and brain are tremendous vessels that are constantly working and changing in all that we do. With more scientific research, I know we can find better and more empathetic ways of treating TBI patients in the short and long term.

It is my sincere hope that I can inspire someone with TBI and their caregivers, family, and friends to treat each other with more compassion and empathy. Just like in life, TBIs will not be overcome with a sprint to the finish; it's a marathon journey with many hills to climb. Trusting your gut instincts, being patient, and giving others the benefit of doubt will go a long way in recovery. While things will never be the same, with some time, you can learn to embrace the difference.

Imagination

18

Life is either a daring adventure, or nothing.

—Helen Keller, activist

What is now proved was once only imagined.

—William Blake, poet

In the 15 years since my accident, I have had the opportunity to ask myself if I have any regrets about having experienced a traumatic brain injury. The accident itself is a tragedy, and that cannot be denied. However, how I have grown and shaped my life since then is precious to me. If I didn't have my TBI, then I imagine I would have to erase the past 15 years, and why would I want to do that? What would be lost instead?

Although I could have dwelled upon what TBI suddenly took away from me, it also cleared the way and opened my life to other greater possibilities. As Mizuta Masahide, the seventeenth-century Japanese poet and samurai, wrote, "My barn having burned down, I can now see the moon." I can now see and appreciate more of life and the human experience. Without my TBI, I may not have stopped and taken stock of all of my blessings and gifts. As you may recall, the first thing I did when I awoke from coma was smile, almost too much! Now I know (I think), I was thankful to be alive and see my family.

For my and Carlos's 60th birthday, we decided to throw a joint party with *exactly* 60 of our friends and family. It was a bittersweet but joyous celebration of two milestones, since it also marked the 10-year point in my recovery. Our sons made purple (my favorite color) tee shirts with our photos on them, and I was able to cook with Michael and Eric as adults, which was so special. Eric not only filmed but also helped arrange for some of his musician friends to perform (Fig 18.1).

Traumatic events have a way of forcing us to take stock of what and who is important to us. They also strip away some of the day-to-day distractions and

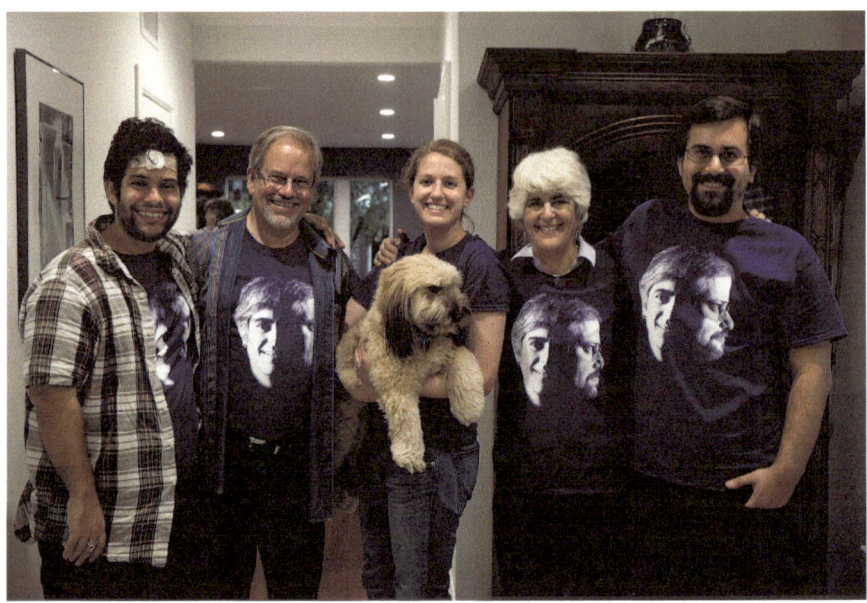

Fig. 18.1 A joyous celebration of 10 years of recovery and our joint 60th birthdays—Eric, Carlos, Sarah, Sunny, me, and Mike

excuses we might normally have. It seems especially poignant that the globe is dealing with a pandemic at the time of this writing. COVID-19 is a highly transmittable, cold- or flu-like respiratory, vascular, gastrointestinal disease, and there is still much we do not know in the medical community about how it is spread among us or operates within the body. What we do know is that it appears asymptomatic in some people and yet ravages others, shutting down their lungs and other organs rapidly and creating "brain fog." The death toll has been immense worldwide, and countries have been in some state of lockdown and quarantine for many months. We are now using new terms such as "self-quarantine" and "social distancing," and in many states and cities, it is now mandatory to wear a mask in public. Although it is still too soon to draw conclusions, COVID-19 shares some eerie similarities with TBI. It appears somewhat random; it can happen to anyone, anywhere, and without warning. Some may recover from COVID-19 in a few weeks or months, while others perish quickly or are left with long-term deficits. In addition, the fear and uncertainty that comes from being unsure of what will happen to ourselves or our loved ones reminds me of those first difficult months of my own recovery.

Therefore, it strikes me that COVID-19 is yet another traumatic life event that can challenge our brain/mind at its core, just like TBI. While TBIs are not contagious, they have profound ripple effects on those around us and require much willpower and support to overcome.

It only makes sense that I would turn to my own disciplines in science and psychiatry to understand what COVID-19 and social isolation are doing to human beings who are social animals by nature. As all of our activities have moved online, telemedicine and teletherapy have become necessary outlets. As a psychiatrist, I know we will be bearing the brunt of COVID-19 for years to come. There will be profound psychological effects and issues for us all, and therapists will be the backbone of helping us through that healing process.

As a psychiatrist specializing in the mind and emotions, you might think that we don't need hard science to help our patients. However, how many times have my OCD patients said to me, "I know it doesn't make sense, it's all in my head but I can't stop feeling anxious unless I do my rituals, my compulsions"? And my course of treatment, whether it involves medications or cognitive behavioral therapy, doesn't just alter their mind, but it changes the function of their brain. It's easy to dismiss mental illness and the mind by saying it's *only* in your head. However, is there any more complex organ in the body than the brain? No! While we can transplant a heart, kidney, lung, and even part of a liver, I can't give you a new brain. You're just lucky to have the one you have. Therefore, let's continue to have your brain work for you. Luckily, it can repair itself in many ways, sometimes using the same neurocircuitry it has before and sometimes by adopting or adapting other neural pathways. When I was recovering from TBI as you have read, it wasn't just with pharmacology and rehabilitative therapy that I got well and have stayed well but by changing my behaviors and thinking about how my emotions were affecting what I did and how I did it.

Therefore, no matter what happens in life, we must be resilient. Authors of the book *Resilient* Hanson and Hanson have described resilience as "determination, the steadfastness and fortitude to endure, cope and survive." They say that resilience is more than managing stress and pain and recovering from trauma; it is about pursuing opportunities in the face of a challenge. Adriana Feder in *Biological Psychology* similarly wrote, "Resilience is the ability to adapt successfully to adversity" (2019). She goes on to say that "At the core of resilience are stress response that are sufficient but not excessive, as well as rapid and efficient psychobiological recovery following stress... Physical exercise can also help buffer the impact of stress by increasing positive mood and neural plasticity in the dopaminergic brain reward circuit."

I can't help but to think that the resilience I tapped into while recovering from my TBI is not that different from the skills that all of us will need to use to recover from COVID-19 both physically and mentally. On a chemical level, when we increase the release of dopamine and bind it to dopamine receptors, we are resilient. We are not all born with the same number of dopamine receptors in our brain, so some of us may need to stimulate the receptors we have with more dopamine to turn on our "motivational circuits," which leads to our resilience. The good news is that turning on more dopamine release to connect to our dopamine receptors is a teachable skill. It comes by learning to pace yourself and to experience positive situations and desires. In a sense, it comes from being positive and not negative when you look at the world. Malcolm Forbes is quoted as saying, "Too many people overvalue what they are not and undervalue what they are." Even when things seem uncertain and overwhelming like COVID-19 (or my TBI), you can choose to put a positive attitude to them. When we lose, we gain at the same time.

Before my accident, I was a prolific cook, making dinner for friends and family and often experimenting with new recipes. While being stuck in self-isolation, I returned to the habit of cooking every night like when the kids were young. Instead of making my signature dishes two times a week, it's given me new inspiration to make something new every night. It has also provided an excuse to again cook with my boys. Through Zoom and Skype sessions, we traded recipes and compared the results. A few weeks in, during a Zoom with Eric, I made one of his favorite childhood desserts, Oreo Cookie cake. I made two "loaves" and put one in the freezer for us to share with Eric when we are done with social distancing. On week 16, he finally gave up his apartment in Manhattan and joined us at our home in Huntington and our first dessert together?! You guessed it, that Oreo cake!

I have always tried to be a force for change. So perhaps it is not so unusual that I would see my brain injury as just another excuse to promote change. However, it's different. Before inciting change was just a part of my mission as a doctor and a teacher to help teach other clinicians or patients. I would draw upon empathy for the insight into what others were experiencing either because of their mental or physical illness or their circumstances, whether they were the same or different from my own. However, for the first time in a very global way, I can understand and empathize with those who have experienced TBI. However, I am lucky enough to still help them not just as a compatriot but as a doctor too.

I have taken up brain injury as a special focus and have contacted colleagues and TBI experts to get advice and learn more. Although my grand round lectures have been postponed or moved to Zoom due to the recent COVID-19 pandemic, it reminds me that in uncertain times, we can still use those resources available to you to continue to learn and grow. It seems not so dissimilar to overcoming TBI. Whether we are fighting health challenges or trying to prevent further harm by self isolating or avoiding activities, there are parallels that we all can relate to.

This quote from author Peter Drucker gives me inspiration:

The best way to predict the future is to create it.

Up to now I have written mostly about what I have lost and what I have done to regain it or repurpose with other resources I didn't lose. However, I feel compelled to end this story of my recovery on a different note. We all have dreams. We all have the woulda, coulda, shoulda moments throughout our life. Sometimes they just remain dreams, and sometimes we get to them later, like my mother who was a fashion designer out of high school and Fashion Institute of Technology (FIT) but then finished her college degree to become a photographer in her 40s. TBI shouldn't prevent us from pursuing our dreams either! However, so many times when I hear or read about those with TBI, it is only about what they lost, what they can't do that they could do before, and how those around them and they themselves have to tolerate what is not the same and how they are different. Different isn't bad and dreams do not have to be lost. That is what TBI has taught me. Yes, I have found workarounds for just about all I could do before. However, I cook without smelling, I walk in springtime and can hear some of the birds but can't smell the flowers, and I trip over the speed bumps pretty regularly. But I value what I *can* do so much more. I take so much more pleasure in teaching others the things I used to do automatically, like how to roll a snickerdoodle ball in cinnamon and sugar and showing them what to look, rather than smell, for when it is done. I remember how hard it is as a doctor and a patient to learn about a new illness that you knew little or nothing about like TBI and realize once again what I've reminded every student and patient, "You truly know you have learned something when you can teach it to someone else!"

No matter your age, new deficits or surprises lie ahead, and they can derail or inspire you and those around you. It's the fiber of the human spirit, our nerve, that teaches us to keep trying and not give up.

Appendix

References and Resources

1. THE EXECUTIVE BRAIN: Frontal Lobes and the Civilized Mind by Dr. Elkhonon Goldberg.
2. http://topachievement.com/smart.html.
3. Here's another one specific for TBI, which was 4 steps: http://www.bist.ca/goal-setting-after-a-brain-injury/.
4. https://www.ncbi.nlm.nih.gov/pmc/articles/PMC1442192/.
5. https://money.cnn.com/2018/05/22/pf/emergency-expenses-household-finances/index.html.
6. https://www.brainandspinalcord.org/medical-expenses-traumatic-brain-injury/.
7. https://www.brainline.org/article/aging-after-brain-injury-brainline-talks-dr-steven-flanagan?page=1.
8. Traumatic brain injury. (n.d.). https://www.asha.org/public/speech/disorders/TBI/.
9. TBI: Get the facts. (2016, April 6). https://www.cdc.gov/traumaticbraininjury/get_the_facts.html.
10. Traumatic brain injury information page. (n.d.). https://www.ninds.nih.gov/disorders/All-Disorders/Traumatic-Brain-Injury-Information-Page.

Books We Mention (or Read)

1. *In an Instant*, Lee and Bob Woodruff.
2. *Over My Head,* Claudia Osborn.
3. *Stroke of Insight,* Jill Bolte Taylor.
4. *The Man Who Mistook His Wife for a Hat*, Oliver Sacks.
5. *An Unquiet Mind*, Kay Redfield Jamison, PhD.
6. *Undercurrents*, Martha Manning, PhD.
7. *The Center Cannot Hold*, Elyn R. Saks, JD.

8. *Metamorphosis, Surviving Brain Injury*, David A. Grant.
9. *I'll Carry the Fork*, Kara L. Swanson.
10. *Resilient*, Rick Hanson, PhD.
11. *Textbook of Traumatic Brain Injury*, edited by Jonathan M. Silver, MD, Thomas W. McAllister, MD, David B. Arciniegas, MD - 3rd edition 2019.

Online Resources

1. www.traumaticbraininjury.com.
2. www.cdc.gov/traumaticbraininjury.
3. National Institute of Neurological Disorders and Stroke. https://www.ninds.nih.gov/Disorders/All-Disorders/Traumatic-Brain-Injury-Information-Page.
4. BrainLine. brainline.org.
5. tbiguide.com.
6. Top 10 TBI blogs. https://www.healthline.com/health/best-traumatic-brain-injury-blogs#1.
7. Brain Injury Association of America. https://www.biausa.org/.
8. Family Caregiver Alliance. https://www.caregiver.org/traumatic-brain-injury.
9. Mayo Clinic. www.mayoclinic.com/health/traumatic-brain-injury.

Glossary

Agonal (breathing) Irregular and ineffective arrhythmic breathing.

Anxiety A temporary or long-term condition in which a person is nervous or apprehensive, anticipating a situation they are uncomfortable about.

Aphasia, acute anomic aphasia The loss of the ability to speak and/or to understand speech. You can have both or just one of these problems. Expressive aphasia is when you can't say what you are trying to say (speech). Receptive aphasia is when you can't understand what people are saying to you. Acute anomic aphasia is a type of expressive aphasia where the patient has trouble naming objects acutely (suddenly).

Arachnoid mater The layer of membrane covering the brain that lies just below the dura mater (*see Figs. 3.1, 3.2, 3.3 chapter 3*).

Autonomic nervous system The "automatic" parts of your nervous system. These nerves control regular functions like heart beating, breathing, and kidney filtering your blood, etc.

Bilateral concussive damage Damage to both right and left sides of your brain, due to trauma (a concussion) to the head.

Bilateral frontal lobes Areas of the brain on both sides of your head, in front of the ears and above the eyes, which involves high cognition or critical thinking.

Cardioversion Shocking the heart to restore normal heartbeat.

Cerebral spinal fluid pressure The fluid that surrounds your brain and spinal cord. The head/skull and spine provide a closed compartment for the fluid to circulate in. This resembles a bottle of sparkling water that is "under pressure." When the bottle is opened, or the skull or spine get penetrated or cracked, like in a TBI, the fluid begins to leak out and the pressure drops. The cerebral spinal fluid (CSF) is clear, and it does NOT look like blood but has some of the same chemicals found in blood.

Chronic small vessel ischemic disease The long-term regular (chronic) loss of blood supply (ischemia) in the small blood vessels.

COVID-19 (COrona Virus Infectious Disease 2019) The novel coronavirus identified first in Wuhan, China, in 2019, which is responsible for a global pandemic.

M. T. Pato, *Nerve*, https://doi.org/10.1007/978-3-031-33433-7

Cranioplasty Surgery in which the skull bone (cranium) is put back together.

Cystic encephalomalacia The softening and/or loss of brain tissue often due to trauma or infection. Cystic implies there can be empty or fluid pockets (cysts).

Disequilibrium The state of being off balance (physical and/or emotional).

Disinhibition The condition, common in TBIs, in which a person is unable to properly regulate or control their behavior or emotions.

Dura mater The outermost layer membrane of the brain, right underneath the skull (*see Figs. 3.1, 3.2, 3.3 chapter 3*).

Edema Swelling.

Gelfilm A synthetic/artificial membrane made to imitate a human membrane like dura mater that was damaged in this case of TBI.

Gliosis Scar tissue in the brain.

Hemicraniectomy Removing half (hemi) the skull bone (cranium).

Hemostasis A procedure to stop (stasis) bleeding (hemo).

Herniation Body tissue protruding through an opening in the tissue/skin and getting squeezed off from blood supply.

Interval involution When an organ or in this case part of the brain shrinks over time.

Intubated/extubated When a patient is in a coma or unable to breath on their own, this procedure puts in breathing tube to the lungs (intubation). Extubation is when the breathing tube is extracted out of the lungs.

Labbe The inferior anastomotic vein on the surface of the brain.

Lacerations Cuts, usually torn and jagged edges.

Left decompressive hemicraniectomy A procedure where the bone is removed from the left side of the skull. The purpose is to allow the injured brain to swell and prevent any further crushing of the brain into the hard skull.

Left temporal lobe The area of the brain over your left ear, which involves language.

Leiomyosarcoma Cancer of the smooth (nonstriated) muscles that are found in many parts of the body including the walls of organs like the uterus, stomach, intestines, and even the lungs.

Malapropism Distortion or misuses of a word, which is often unintentional and sometimes humorous.

Medical coma When medication is used to keep a patient unconscious (coma) to allow them to heal over time. These can be long (months or more) or shorter (in my case, 3 days).

Meninges A general name to refer to the membranes covering the brain and spinal cord (see dura, arachnoid, and pia mater).

Monopolar cautery To burn (cauterize) the end of a blood vessel during surgery to prevent bleeding out.

Musculocutaneous flap The attached muscle (musculo) and skin (cutaneous) on the skull. In surgery, this was the piece (flap) that was not cut out completely but put back over the area where the bone was taken out (*see hemicraniectomy*).

Neuromuscular Related to the nerves, which are attached to muscles.

Neuro-otology evaluation Study of the neurological aspects of the ear. Often involves the examination of hearing and balance.

Nonhemorrhagic shear injuries Damage to brain cells due to tearing of the tissue, which do not leave red dye-like blood stains.

Obsessive compulsive disorder (OCD) A mental condition that involves repetitive thoughts or obsessions and performing acts called compulsions. These can be either physical or mental compulsions in an effort to make the thoughts causing the anxiety go away.

Occult bleeding Bleeding that cannot be easily seen because it is hidden from view through an X-ray, scan, or obscured by another organ (it may become visible later through bruise or staining).

Omentum A membrane that lines the abdomen (belly) below the lungs and diaphragm to help keep all the organs in place (liver, stomach, kidneys, intestines). In brain surgery, it is sometimes a potential storage or "host" site for the portion of skull removed.

Paresis Slight/partial paralysis.

Peripheral hemosiderin staining The red color, kind of like a dye, that blood cells have and when the blood dries on your brain it can leave this red stain.

Periventricular and subcortical white matter Periventricular means in the brain areas near the open part in the brain called the ventricles. The ventricles are open cavities in the brain where the cerebral spinal fluid gathers and circulates.

Pia mater The membrane just under the arachnoid mater (and the space below it) in direct contact with the brain tissue (cerebral cortex) (*see Figs. 3.2, 3.3 chapter 3*).

Post-traumatic stress disorder (PSTD) Experiencing emotional trauma in situations based upon an event that happened in the past (post-traumatic) that made you fearful, anxious, or traumatized the first time.

Punctate white matter foci Little dots/holes that appear as white areas rather than gray areas, of the brain that were traumatized with the concussion. They correspond to small spots where the concussion or trauma caused brain cells to die.

Respiratory rate variability Breathing can change and fluctuate even from minute to minute while you are sitting still, and therefore it can be variable.

Resilience The ability to bounce back and recover. An area of ongoing research within neuroscience.

"Scoop and Run" EMS protocol to "scoop" up the patient by stabilizing the head, neck, and back and then "run" in an ambulance to the nearest hospital.

"Stay and Play" EMS protocol to "stay" at the scene of the accident, stabilize the patient in every way possible, and "play" by performing procedures on the spot before transporting them to the hospital.

Subdural hematoma Blood collecting under the layers of tissue (dura mater, arachnoid mater, pia mater) that surround the brain.

Syncopal episode Fainting spell.

Traumatic brain injury (TBI) An injury to the brain tissue due to a blow to the head or trauma of some sort. Two categories of traumatic brain injury, which I have defined and lectured on, are ssTBI and mmTBI. A single severe TBI (ssTBI) is one single blow or trauma to the brain. A multiple mild TBI (mmTBI) refers to a series of injuries to the brain, such as several concussions. To be clear, I do not think any head trauma can be referred to as mild per se.

Tinnitus A condition of the ear where the person has the sensation of hearing a continuous noise, often of a ringing quality, roaring sound, or a continuous buzz.

Vertigo Dizziness sometimes accompanied by confusion.

Index